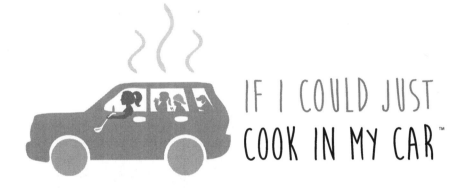

IF I COULD JUST
COOK IN MY CAR™

IF I COULD JUST COOK IN MY CAR

A Busy Mom's Guide to Healthy Family Meals
With Less time, Stress and Money

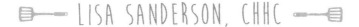 LISA SANDERSON, CHHC

If I Could Just Cook In My Car

The content of this book is for general instruction only. Each person's physical, emotional, and spiritual condition is unique. The instruction in this book is not intended to replace or interupt the reader's relationship with a physician or other professional. Please consult your doctor for matters pertaining to your specific health and diet.

To contact author, visit:
www.enjoyhealthy.me

For my daughters, Emily and Paige,
who I am lucky enough to drive around,
my husband Doug for taking the journey with me
and Gus, my furry child who is the easiest to feed.

Thank you for all your love and support.

GRATEFUL

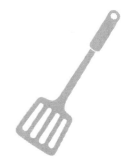

For my husband Doug, who has loved and supported me for a really long time! I cannot begin to thank you for making it possible for me to stay home with the kids and to follow my passion to create my own business and write this book. Love you more...

For Emily and Paige, who have taught me so much about who I am and who I want to be. Thank you for being my best friends and for all of your support, ideas and recipe testing. I am so proud of both of you and know you will succeed at whatever you choose to do.

For Gus, for keeping me company while I wrote this book and always being such a good listener. You had some pretty big paws to fill and you are doing an amazing job. WOOF!

For My Mom and Dad, well because they are my Mom and Dad. I am so lucky to have parents that have always encouraged me to pursue my dreams and supported me along the way.

For Carol, the one person I can talk to, vent to and text when I need support about food stuff. Thanks for always being there and helping me on this Journey.

For Lisa D, I am so glad I found such a great accountability partner and friend. Thank you for being the first one to read this book and assure me that it was worth publishing.

For Lisa B, not sure how I lucked out finding you but I could not have finished this without you. Thank you for making me look good and pushing me to the finish line.

For Kris, who not only did the cover art, but saved me with a totally cool Octopus.

For all my other amazing friends and family, you know who you are, for always being there for me. When it comes to friends I have learned a few things… first quality is much more important than quantity, second "family" does not always mean you have to be related by blood, third it is an added bonus when your friends have awesome vacation homes where you can all make amazing memories, and last a true friend is someone who you know is always there even if they move away or you don't talk to for awhile. I love you all.

For my clients, in school we learn about mirroring which is the idea that we learn about ourselves while working with our clients. With each client I learn so much not just about how to be a better health coach, but also about myself and how to be a better me. Thank you.

TABLE OF CONTENTS

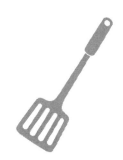

PART 1: THE METHOD

PART 2: TOOLKIT

APPENDIX

INTRODUCTION

Life is funny, isn't it? If you had told me when I was a teenager that at 46 I would be a health coach writing a book about meal planning for busy moms, I would have laughed in your face. (Although, if you had told me I would be running half marathons, I probably would have laughed even harder. So glad I stopped listening to my teenage self!) Truth is I was going to be a movie producer.

After making it to LA, I decided I needed to get my MBA focusing on International Business. That way I would be better prepared to conquer the film business where there was an increase in international investors at the time (and I'd also be better qualified to walk a famous person's dog as an entry level job to break into the business). That led to coming back to the East Coast to get my MBA at Georgetown, getting married, switching to marketing (because launching a toilet bowl cleaner is a lot like making a movie—oh, the things we can convince ourselves!) and then getting pregnant.

I found out I was pregnant the day I was interviewing for a new job, since I was unhappy with my old one. Not wanting to start a new job with an infant at home, I decided not go back to work after my daughter was born. Transitioning to not working was hard. I needed to feel needed and busy so I got involved. I joined the nursery school committee and eventually became chair, helped to launch a new camp at nursery school, I was class mom, PTO president, and volunteered for everything. Soon with two daughters, I had transitioned to being a "full-time mom," with not a lot of time to focus on myself.

When your kids are young they need a lot of attention, their needs are primarily physical and they need to be supervised at all times. As they get older, the physical needs are more basic and not as demanding—needing rides, food, clothing, electronics—and become more emotional—middle school girls are mean, boys are bullies and hormones wreak havoc. But the good news is, more time for you since they are at school more and you can leave them unsupervised for a bit without as much worry they will put their fingers in outlets.

I loved being involved in their schools and activities, but I began to realize I needed more. When my kids were finally both in school, I started going to the gym more and paying more attention to me. I made some significant changes in my diet and lifestyle. It had such a positive impact on my life. I knew I wanted to show others that they could ENJOY HEALTHY too! (Yeah, that's where my company name came from.) I became certified to teach Zumba, then Pilates mat and then to do group fitness training. Just as I was completing those certifications, I stumbled onto Health Coaching and it just made perfect sense. I enrolled in the Institute of Integrative Nutrition, and never taught an exercise class (OK, I did teach one and realized it was not for me.)

I knew I had found my "calling" with health coaching. When I was trying to come up with a name for my business, I really wanted something that reflected my belief that living a healthy lifestyle doesn't have to be a chore—you can ENJOY HEALTHY! It was really that easy.

Being healthy doesn't mean deprivation and pain—you can enjoy yummy food, not being tired, being fit and looking great. It wasn't until working on my business cards that I realized the word "joy" in ENJOY HEALTHY, and in my name. My middle name is JOY. It's ironic, because I did not always consider myself a very joyful person, but that all changed when I started living a healthier lifestyle and even more when I started sharing what I know with others and helping them to live healthier lives. My work gives me joy.

One day I was on a longer training run (where I do my best thinking), I pondered what I was going to cook that week. In thinking through my family's calendar for the week, I realized that I would be spending most of my afternoons in the car driving my kids around. I thought, "If I could just cook in my car"... and that is where the idea for the book came from. I want to help other moms figure out how to feed their families healthy meals even with hectic schedules!

My focus has always been Busy Moms. I am one myself and I get it. The frantic pace of life can be a struggle; we not only have to take care of ourselves, but also be the one who is responsible for our family as well. My goal was to help make the eating healthy part easy and convenient so that you have more time and energy. The concepts for eating healthy aren't hard, and I show you how to fit the "effort" part into your already jam-packed life. It becomes routine, it gets easier and the time spent is worth the decrease in stress. You and your family will eat better and you really will feel better!

Are you ready to ENJOY HEALTHY? Let's do it!

PART 1: THE METHOD

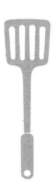

CHAPTER 1

THE TOUGHEST JOB IN THE WORLD

It is true, being a parent is the toughest job in the world. Look at the job description.

ALL TIME CARE GIVER

Lifetime, 24-hour 7-day-a-week position. Early in your career be prepared to go without sleep, grooming, self care or food. You will be on constant call when your boss needs you to feed them, help them with hygiene, or to soothe them when they are just not happy. Will be responsible for training in social etiquette and proper self-care. Although later in career the personal care and supervision responsibilities will decrease, you will add the jobs of counselor, and enforcer—good nagging skills may be necessary in order to make sure that the Boss stays on track. Good scheduling and logistic skills a must. Will also have added jobs of Chauffeur, Chef, Maid, and personal shopper.

Although, for most, day-to-day demands decrease after 18 years, constant concern will continue and you need to be on call for any needs/crisis that arise.

Note: Possibility of reporting to an additional boss or bosses during career, starting at beginning with each one.

And we took this job willingly! Okay, so this job description is lacking the benefits; let's take a look at those.

> *Benefits*: No monetary pay. Compensation will be in the form of hugs, kisses, love and a sense of overwhelming pride when Boss succeeds.

We all know that it is worth it. Especially when we hear their first word, see them take their first step, watch them perform on stage or on the field, receive that diploma and most of all when they say "I love you!"

• Stay at home vs working parent... •

I never thought that I would be a "stay at home mom." Remember I was going to be a movie producer. Kids were never really on my radar. Even when I changed career paths and went into marketing, I was going to keep working after my first child. But life has a funny way of throwing you curve balls to put you on the path you were meant to take—mine was finding out I was pregnant the day I was interviewing for a new job. Not wanting to start a new job pregnant, I stayed at my current job, vested in my 401K and then decided to stay home with my daughter.

Getting involved in my children's schools and activities and taking on volunteer part-time jobs kept my brain working. The women I worked with on these committees were just like me, usually with multiple degrees and trying to figure out how they ended up taking care of kids instead of major clients. They tried to balance their kids' needs as well as their own, but often the scales would swing to the side of the kids. The working parents I knew also struggled. Torn between working, caring for their kids, trying to be involved in their kid's school and activities and time for themselves.

Whether you stay at home or work outside the home, the responsibilities are the same. We are responsible for making sure that these creatures we brought into our family are happy, healthy and safe. When one of these basic needs are not met, we feel guilty and do our best to fix it if possible.

We all want the best for our kids. We all try our best and we all feel that we fail at some time in some way, but I try to remember that my parents probably felt that way also and I turned out OK—hopefully my kids will too! The best I can do is my best and to try to provide them with love, support and tools to help them succeed. And every once in a while, they will say or do something that makes me realize they have been listening, like when my daughter said she thought maybe she would try eliminating dairy and/or gluten because she has been really congested lately. Yes, this is my segue into what I really want to talk about—feeding our kids.

After all, this is the busy mom's guide to feeding her family healthy meals with less time, stress and money. When you and your family start eating better, your energy goes up and life as a whole just feels better. Trust me, it's true! I know you don't have a lot of time so let's get right to it. And let's go back to that job description.

· Job Requirement: Must be able · to provide all meals and snacks

As a health coach, I often start working with a client who comes to me because she wants to lose weight, get rid of sugar cravings, or have more energy, but we end up spending a lot of our time together figuring out what she is going to feed her family. Let's face it—the looming "what are we going to eat" is forever there and is not only stressful but also frustrating. You have to be a meal planner, shopper and cook, all while making sure that you are providing food that will properly nourish your kids' growing bodies.

When working with clients, I try not to lose sight of their individual needs and goals as well. Everyone in the family should be considered when making meal choices, most importantly the one preparing the meal should prepare food they want to eat and not have to be a short order chef. By the time you finish this short book you will know all about meal planning and how including your family in the process will ease kitchen chaos.

This book has two simple goals. The first is to introduce you to my **ADD, AWARE, ADJUST, ENJOY**™ strategy for feeding your family. This strategy provides an approach for transitioning your family to eating real, healthy food. The second goal is to help you implement this strategy and set you up for long term success by taking you step by step through a meal planning process. I provide you with tools and suggestions that will allow you to have less stress, while saving money and time.

Just a note, there is no magic pill when it comes to achieving your and your family's health goals; if there were, everyone would be healthy. There is also no "one size fits all" kind of plan. Everyone is different in their likes, dislikes, genetics, and lifestyle, so it sometimes takes trying different things to figure out what works. The concepts required to ENJOY HEALTHY are not difficult, but they do take a little effort—more so in the beginning as you are figuring it out. The effort is worth it, and it will become less time consuming as you become familiar with the process. For example, in the beginning you might have to do a lot of label reading, but as you learn which products are a better choice, you will spend less time doing the exploratory research. Same with meal planning. In the beginning it may take a while to build your go-to meal idea list, but once in place, it will make meal planning a breeze.

My process will ultimately save time, reduce stress and maybe even reduce your grocery bills. More importantly, you and your family will be able to ENJOY HEALTHY and you will be teaching your kids the important skills they need to live a healthy life.

· Three Principles ·

Three underlying theories guide my health coaching approach. The first I already spoke about, the fact that we are all different and need to find what works best for our families and us. There is no one program, diet, exercise, food, etc that works for everyone and every family. That is why there are thousands of books in the health and wellness section and hours of television shows each day with segments on the latest diet trend. Each plan works for some people. The challenging part in the beginning is figuring out what works for you!

There will be some trial and error to figure out what will work with your family, but trust me it does get easier. It is the same as learning anything new. After you get through the initial learning curve, it becomes much more intuitive. The results are less stress about if you are feeding your family healthy, less time with daily meal prep and at the grocery store, and hopefully savings on your food bills.

The second principle is a quote I borrow from Micheal Pollan's book *In Defense of Food*. "Eat food. Not too much. Mostly plants." (I like to say, "Eat real food, mainly plants, not too much!) It is amazing to me how simple it can really be. Eat real food, food that comes from a plant, not made in a plant. Eat food that was put on this earth by nature (or the higher being you might believe in) not by another human who created it in a laboratory. Later I will talk more about becoming AWARE of what you are eating and give you help on determining where your food is coming from and guide you toward "real food."

When people hear the "mainly plants" part, they get a little nervous—"I don't want to be a vegetarian or vegan." Eating mainly plants does not mean you have to eliminate all animal products. For some, that might be the right choice, and personally I find eating a mainly plant based diet, with some fish, is the right choice for me. The rest of my family still eats meat on occasion (and no, I don't cook twice each night! More on this later.) The idea is that we should be focusing on the plants we eat, not the animal portion of our diet. This will be discussed further in the ADJUST section, when I help you change your mindset about meal planning. It doesn't mean stop eating animal products, it means eat more plants. As I said, "Eat real food, mainly plants, not too much."

"Not too much" - this is not just for those trying to lose weight. Understanding *how much* we need to eat to feel our best is as important as knowing *what* we need to eat. I never dwell on calories or serving sizes, because when you are eating real food it just works itself out. Your body tells you what it needs and how much—you just need to listen.

The third principle I teach is one that struck me after listening to a lecture. The speaker said to focus on the good food that should be added. It really hit me that we focus so much on what we should not eat and I want to focus on what we can and should eat, to really ENJOY HEALTHY.

From there I created **ADD, AWARE, ADJUST, ENJOY**™! First we focus on the ADD, the things you should be doing and how to ADD those things into your diet and lifestyle. The next step is to become AWARE of what you are currently doing so you can ADJUST (make minor changes). In the AWARE section, you discover what you should be looking for on labels and in recipes; often we don't even realize what is really in our food. Once we are AWARE, it is easy to ADJUST by making small changes.

Now let's take a closer look at the **ADD, AWARE, ADJUST, ENJOY**™ method!

CHAPTER 2

ADD

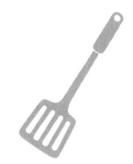

Step One is focusing on the ADD. We learn about this in parenting books and lectures, right? Focus on the positive; reinforce the behavior we want to see. Doing this not only teaches us what to do, but often when focusing on the ADD, we tend to crowd out some of the not so good.

Let me explain using my first ADD, drinking water.

· Water ·

We all know that drinking water is good for us. Whenever my kids don't feel well, or have a headache, I tell them to drink water. You hear it all the time: "Are you drinking enough water?"

Our bodies are made up mainly of water. Replenishing the water our body uses in daily function as well as the excess we might use to sweat is really important. Drinking enough water helps everything in our body from making our skin look better, to helping things "move along" if you get my drift. Yet most people struggle with drinking enough, me included!

I am sure you have heard that you should drink 8 glasses of water a day; or take your body weight in pounds and divide it in half, and drink that much water in ounces per day; or drink between ½ oz to 1 oz per pound you weigh. These are all guidelines. Like everything else, you need to figure out what amount is best for you! I like to use the pee test—I know, gross, but it works. Your pee should be a light yellow (think lemonade) color. If it is darker, you need more water. If it is clear, you may be drinking too much (and yes, you can drink too much water!)

People also ask, what counts as water—well, water counts as water. Water with lemon counts—or infused with some other fruits or vegetables; herbal tea counts (not decaffeinated, but herbal tea without caffeine). For those just starting off that are struggling with water, maybe some seltzer without artificial or natural sweeteners in moderation to start. Ideally, we don't want to include seltzer as our primary water since it is actually acid forming in the body (not a concept I am going to go into here, but just know it is not great for you in large quantities), but sometimes when you are making a switch you need a crutch and if you need to drink seltzer to help you transition to drinking more water, go for it.

Now let's apply the ADD principle. Drinking water is my #1 ADD. It is the first thing I tell every client, first piece of advice I give at every lecture, and the first action step in this book!

Commit to drink more water, and give your kids more water. Get a reusable water bottle for you and your kids. Fill theirs and put it in their lunch boxes. Fill yours and carry it with you. When you are out to eat, order water. When you think you might be hungry, drink some water first to make sure you are not just thirsty. When you are about to drink another cup of coffee, drink a cup of hot water first.

With all this ADDing, you are actually crowding out some of the things that aren't as good for your health goals. You are giving your kids water for lunch instead of juice boxes; you are ordering water instead of soda at dinner; you are drinking water before you eat thus maybe avoiding an unneeded snack or reducing the amount you eat; you are substituting water for coffee thus reducing your coffee and caffeine. Never did I say to not drink juice, soda, or coffee, it just happens by focusing on the ADD.

By the way, I did sneak in some tricks there that I want to point out. You should get reusable water bottles as it really does help to keep track of how much water you drink. I find the straw kind helps me drink more. My bottle is always with me, so it is easy to sip on during my busy day. Just make sure that you clean your bottles thoroughly and on a regular basis. There are also apps you can put on your phone to keep track and remind you to drink—these can be fun for you and your kids.

Sipping hot water is a great way to ADD. I find that a lot of the time when people reach for the hot cup of coffee or tea it is more about drinking something warm and soothing than the caffeine. Sounds weird, but try hot water—I did and now I actually crave it.

I know what you are thinking, how am I going to get my kids to drink more water? First of all, your kids should be taking water for lunch and it should be the first option for drinks at home or out. Give them a glass in the morning before they go to school, and send them to school with a water bottle to keep on their desk (most schools will allow this is if it just water). Keep a jug in the refrigerator that is infused with fruit like watermelon, oranges, or lemons, or vegetables like cucumber. Let them experiment and figure out what they like! Then take those infused waters and freeze them to add to water or to eat as ice pops in the summer. I am not saying that your kids can never drink anything else, just have water be their go-to drink and have other things be occasional. To help them transition, you can add water to their favorite juice or other beverage gradually changing the ratio until it is mostly water with just a splash of the other.

Send your kids with water to sporting events instead of Gatorade. Or send with both, or watered down Gatorade. Kids that play sports really hard may need to replenish electrolytes, etc.

with Gatorade or a sport replacement drink but water works well for the majority of kids (and adults). And as an aside, if your kid is playing competitive enough that they need a sport replacement drink or you or your kids are participating in endurance activities or they are playing for long periods of time (like a tournament), consider something besides highly artificial Gatorade, especially if they are drinking it a lot. It is easy to make your own sport recovery drink using salt, sugar and water. Using water as the base, flavor with lemon juice or other real fruit juices, and sweeten with honey or maple syrup, and then add salt. But as you see, the base is still water.

As with a lot of the ADDs, make it fun for the little kids. If you can start them drinking water early, you will be teaching them one of the most important healthy habits anyone can have. My girls are avid water drinkers and will ask for it first before anything else because it has always been the go-to in our house. Before we had a water cooler, we either had a refrigerator with a water dispenser in the door or a pitcher of filtered water in the refrigerator.

Remember water is not just in the form of the water we drink, water is also in food like fruits and vegetables, which actually leads us to our next ADD.

· Fruits and Vegetables ·

The next ADD is fruits and vegetables, especially green leafy vegetables. No brainer, right? You knew it was coming.

ADD in fruits and vegetables, especially leafy green veggies. Yes, I know what you are thinking. How do you expect me to get my kids to eat more veggies, especially the green ones? Well, I understand and I went through ups and downs with my kids eating fruits and veggies as well. I came up with this little rule of thumb/trick that helps me, my kids and my clients and their kids, eat more fruits and veggies.

Every time you sit down to eat a meal or think about having a snack, try to eat a fruit or a vegetable as part of it. If your kids want nachos for a snack, that is fine, but make sure you at least offer salsa and/or guacamole with it. By offer, I mean put it out in front of them. If you are making pizza, put a little extra sauce on or maybe add veggies as a topping, like cut up broccoli or mushrooms. It's OK if you start with just a few and then add more later. My kids actually prefer pizza with broccoli and black olives now to plain or any meat.

Offer apple and peanut butter for a snack, chips with veggies and hummus or dressing. Make sure there is always a fruit or veggie in their lunch boxes or even on their breakfast plate. Even if it is not always eaten, it is training them that ever time we eat, we eat a fruit or vegetable. Of course trying new things is great, but if you find a few options they like, it is fine, especially in the beginning to use them over and over. The point is for them to get into this healthy habit of including more fruits and vegetables in their diets. Later you can work on expanding the offerings so they are "eating a rainbow," a diet that includes fruits and vegetable that are all the colors of the rainbow.

One way to help ADD fruits and veggies is to offer veg soups, salads or even fruit before a meal. I remember growing up we often had half a grapefruit before dinner. By offering your kids fruit or a salad before dinner every night, you are training them with this great behavior, one that maybe they won't adopt right away, but may later like when they are off at college or after. My kids actually told me they ate salad every day at camp (yes I believe them!) because they are so used to eating it at home. And yes, if for now, the only way they will eat vegetables or salad is with a not ideal dressing, that is fine. When we talk about AWARE and ADJUST, we can work on finding better choices; for now just get them to eat the green stuff!

Of course we want to get our kids to eat more fruits and vegetables, but we should be eating them too! Eating a salad or a vegetable soup before a meal is not only a great way to increase your plant intake, but you may also find you are eating less of other foods. This is not only about weight loss, but by eating foods with greater nutritional density, like fruits and veggies, you might "crowd out" foods that may not be such nutritional power-houses. In the AWARE section, we will talk about having a different mindset about how we look at our meals. Make the vegetables the stars and the grains, and if you choose, animal proteins, the supporting players.

You may be thinking this all sounds great and these are good ideas, but your kids are not going to convert easily. First of all, remember this is a process. You don't have to start serving kale at every meal on day one. Small steps are fine. Start with more fruit, maybe try a new vegetable or incorporating a new vegetable every so often. I have learned the hard way, that it is often best to have a back up if you are trying something new. If you are serving asparagus for the first time, maybe also have some broccoli as an option if you know they like that.

Also, make the stuff taste good. Maybe put some cheese on the broccoli, let them dip veggies in dressing or make a stir fry with tons of veggies and chicken or shrimp and teriyaki sauce. You can use training wheels. It would be great if everyone loved every vegetable raw, steamed or sauteed by itself, but that may not happen right away. Eventually it is great if you and your family learn to love the flavors of the fruit or veggies by themselves and you don't have to enhance the flavors, but this might not ever happen. I still have to "mask" the flavors of some things for my husband!

Take it slow and don't send anyone into shock by completely overhauling your kitchen (unless of course you are up for the challenge and then go for it!) There are ways to ease the transition in less obvious (and potentially fun) ways. One way is to "hide" the vegetables. Although this doesn't really help to teach kids about eating more vegetables at first, it can help them ease into the idea, especially younger kids, although sometimes the older ones may be harder to convert. Adding additional pureed or chopped veggies to spaghetti sauce, or using puree in baking, or making a pureed soup where no one is really sure what is in it are all ways to "trick" the mind into not realizing what vegetables you are eating.

Along these lines are smoothies. Smoothies are great for getting lots of different fruits and vegetables into our diet. There is a reason they are so popular and you see so much information about them. They are a really easy way to ADD lots of great stuff into your diet! There are lots of smoothie recipes out there, but its also fun and easy to create your own. Play with different combinations of bases (coconut water, non dairy milks, juices) and different fruits and veggies. When you are ready, this is a great place to add in some super foods or protein sources—chia seeds, flax seed (ground), cinnamon, hemp seeds, almond butter, coconut oil. Your kids (or husband!) will never know. (Check the appendix for my smoothie guide including some recipes.)

Experiment with different bases and fruits to find one that you and/or your kids like. Then add in the "harder" stuff, like green leafy vegetables. You can make it a game or a science experiment. Start with a base fruit smoothie you know the kids like, maybe banana, strawberry with almond milk. Then add in one leaf of kale (or spinach since it is milder) and taste it; next time add in two leaves, and then three; continue until they tell you that it has changed the taste too much. As you do this experiment you can have them track it on paper, noticing the changes in color, texture and taste. If you like to juice and have a juicer, you can do the same type of experiment starting with fruit juice or sweet veggies and then ADD the not as sweet veggies to taste. Except for the color change, it may not taste that different.

Little kids often enjoy the fun colors, like the green goop or the blood "beet" juice.

Get your kids involved! Take your kids with you to the farmer's market or to the grocery store and get them to pick out fruits and veggies. With younger kids (or if your older ones are up for it), it is fun to take them and ask them to pick one new fruit or vegetable a week. We are so lucky to live in a time when we have instant access at our fingertips to information about a new food, how to prepare it and recipes. We don't have to look through tons of cook books, we just need a computer, or we can even do research on our phones in the stores! (Whole Foods has wifi and I am sure other stores do too.) So don't be afraid, if your kid thinks a star fruit looks really cool it is a small investment to try it. Your kids can go home, look it up online and figure out where it comes from and how you eat it.

The tricks here for getting your little kids to ADD fruits and vegetables work for adults in the house and the older kids, too. Remember that you are a role model, and your attitude toward these changes will influence your kids' acceptance.

As part of this ADD, I mentioned trying to ADD green leafy vegetables. These veggies are high in many vitamins and minerals including calcium, magnesium, iron, potassium, and vitamins A, C, E and K. They are loaded with fiber, folic acid, chlorophyll and lots of other really good stuff! They truly are nutritional superstars. But they are one of the harder vegetables to ADD for some who are not used to them. I talked about sneaking them into smoothies, masking them with sauce or adding them into stir fry, but there are some family friendly ways I have found to actually get the kids to eat them.

Keep an open mind, but my number one recommendation for getting anyone to eat more green leafy vegetables is Kale Chips! We have all heard about kale. Well, kale chips are an easy, fun way to introduce anyone to this superstar. I actually give all of my clients a kale sample and tell them to make chips for their families, and the reports are almost always positive. Often times the only problem is that because, like most greens, kale shrinks up when cooked, and there isn't enough when you make just one bunch! I have included the recipe with other favorite recipes in the appendix. There are many variations of how to cook kale chips if you search the Internet. Be creative with toppings. I have had them both sweet and savory and they are yummy both ways. They are super fun to eat if you are patient and get the texture right, not soggy but not burnt.

Other ideas for greens are to use them for wraps. This can be as simple as making lettuce wraps or you can steam collard greens and use them to make wraps as well. Replace bread, flour wraps, tortillas or taco shells with lettuce or greens. Just make sure to use a heartier green so it doesn't fall apart!

Okay, It's time to take a break and get up off your chair and stretch. Which leads directly to my next ADD.

· Movement ·

My next ADD is movement. Now I know that has nothing to do with feeding our families, but it does have a big part to do with keeping our families healthy. We all have heard and know how important it is for us to move our bodies. I like to use movement instead of exercise, because the word exercise sometimes scares people off. Also, exercise implies a planned activity, and movement just means that.

If you are already moving, by having an exercise routine or if your kids play sports or do some other regularly activity, that is great! But if you do not currently actively incorporate movement into your or your kids' lives, this is a very important ADD.

Movement does not have to mean going to the gym or getting your kids out on the field. It can simply be taking a walk, or playing on a swing set. More and more we are hearing that we don't have to get our "exercise" in one chunk. It counts if you do 10 minutes, 3 times a day. Walk the dog or go outside with the dog and your kids and kick the ball around, park farther from the mall or store, walk to school with your kids if you can—you get the added benefit of the extra mileage since you get to walk home too, or just put on some great music and dance around your house with or without your kids. Just get your heart pumping and your body moving.

You can try to make some new rules in your house. In my house, I tried to institute the rule that if you want to watch TV, homework needs to be done and while you are watching you need to walk on the treadmill, do some stretching or static exercises. (No, it didn't work that well, but I will say my teenager just joined my gym and I think it is so she can watch TV at night while she is on the machines there—she doesn't like our treadmill.) I know this is pretty extreme, but maybe it can be something as easy as giving the kids responsibility for walking the dog, raking the leaves, shoveling the snow or pushing the vacuum. One push back I get from my kids is "you haven't been in school all day, we just need a rest." My response is "yeah I haven't been sitting at a desk all day, so go outside and walk around the block and get some fresh air or ride your bike, kick a ball or if you can't go outside, move a little." Inside dancing is always fun and there are even video games now that get you moving. (My younger daughter loves to Hula Hoop. While she is challenging herself to see how long she can keep the hoop up or what tricks she can do without dropping it, she isn't thinking about how great this is for her very important core muscles!)

Now kids do have gym class a few days a week, which is great because at least they get to move around a little. We should all have gym class that makes us move. Get in the habit of moving and making conscious movement a part of your routine. Remember simple things count. If we are sitting at a desk or sitting in our cars all the time driving our kids around, we need to ADD movement to not only keep our bodies healthy, but to avoid the aches and pains that being in those sitting, hunched over positions for long periods of time can sometimes cause.

Kids often play sports or organized activities like dance or martial arts. What about you? Get yourself moving. If you are not going to do it for yourself, do it for your kids. Teaching them the importance of keeping our bodies strong and physically fit is important. Take some time to think about how you can ADD movement into your family's lives. Maybe you plan a family bicycle ride or hike, go outside and play ball, push your child on the swing or just take the dog for the walk around the block together. It is not only beneficial for keeping your bodies healthy, but it is great for your mental well-being and moods as well.

· Meal Planning ·

Later in the book I have a whole section on meal planning and my meal planning program. Here I just want to discuss why this is such and important ADD.

Benjamin Franklin said, "Failure to plan, is planning to fail." Although I am not sure this is always true, when it comes to feeding our families and ourselves, I really do think it is spot on. Planning reduces stress, can save you time and money and sets you up for success. Yes, planning does involve setting aside time to plan and prep, but the up front work is worth the reward of knowing what is for dinner, or having a healthy option on hand when someone is "starving" and needs to eat! Planning takes away the stress of having to make on the spot decisions, allowing you to make better choices.

I know that it seems like a lot to ask to schedule time to plan, shop and prep. But I can tell you that if you take the time up front, you will save the time later. Plus as I mentioned you get the added benefit of saving money and reducing stress.

Every Saturday, I print out my family's calendar for the next week and I sit down and go through the meal planning process. I determine the "menu," check the pantry and the freezer for what I have on hand and make a shopping list. On Sunday I go to the market, and when it is open the farmer's market, and I do my big shopping for the week. I then come home and I prep for the week. I cook and prep what I can including cleaning and storing my greens and other vegetables so when I need them they are ready. I might cut up a lot of veggies and make a dip for snacking, or make a soup, or cook some greens to have in the refrigerator for a quick lunch. I almost always roast sweet potatoes and some other veggies, and soak and maybe cook the grains I may need for the week. This does take a chunk of time out of my day, but makes things so much easier during the week.

Taking this time to plan and prep really does save time later. It also can save you money since you have a list when you go to the store. Most importantly, it can reduce the amount of stress you have. Do not underestimate the role that stress plays in your health. Study after study shows that stress is a contributing factor to disease. Of course there are physical stressors, like eating the wrong foods, or putting excess stress on certain body parts, but the emotional stress wreaks havoc too and produces the same effect.

Feeding your family is a big responsibility. Not only just the actual act of making sure there is food that everyone likes and will eat available when they need or want it, you need to make sure you are providing food that will fulfill their nutritional requirements and is healthy. Having this one area of your life under control is huge. Parents these days have enough to stress about, not just our kids' health, safety, and the world they are being brought up in, but we have stressful jobs, hobbies, activities and other commitments. It all takes more of a toll than you think. If you are one of the lucky ones that can easily manage your stress, that is great. For the rest of us, meditation and yoga can help, but finding other ways to reduce stress, including meal planning, is really important to overall health and well being.

Meal planning also helps increase the amount of meals we cook at home from scratch! Most people are able to ADD more home cooked fresh meals when they start implementing meal planning and as we will see in the next ADD, home cooked meals are about a lot more than just the food.

· Love ·

I am not a really super touchy feely type of gal. But there are a lot of reasons and ways to ADD love and there is a huge value to your health to focus on this area.

When you are cooking and providing yourself and your family with home cooked meals, there is that extra ingredient— Love. OK, you might say that when you are cooking you are feeling anything but love. Maybe sometimes you are feeling pressure or resentment, but hopefully some of the time you enjoy cooking. And even if you don't enjoy cooking, (actually even more so if you don't enjoy cooking) you are doing it out of love for your family.

Again, you may say that you are doing it out of necessity, but if you didn't want what was best for your family, because you love and care about them, then you wouldn't have picked up this book, and you wouldn't be worried or care about what you are feeding them. Being a parent can be a thankless job! Especially when they are young and living with you. (I now thank my mom all the time for putting up with me and doing all she did, now that I realize all that entailed! Sometimes when my daughters do something or are having emotional/friend issues, I call my mom and say I am sorry—now I get it! But I digress....)

Love is a very powerful ingredient in our meals. It is lacking when we eat out, especially when we eat out at fast food restaurants where a machine made our food. You took the time to plan the meal, shop for the meal taking care to pick each ingredient, you cut every vegetable and cooked every bite. Even if you used some convenience foods or something pre-made, that special ingredient is still in there. So, although they may not appreciate it or seem to appreciate it, your kids are still getting the benefits of it just like the broccoli you hid in the pasta sauce.

Although this isn't a parenting book, I do believe it is important to teach kids to respect and appreciate the food they are cooked. Hopefully they do this automatically after seeing how much time and effort you put into their meals, but you can train them. When you get a chance to eat as a family, maybe they could ask to be excused and at the same time thank you for dinner. (No, you don't have to tell them to say thank you to you, but maybe your spouse could tell them or say it to set an example; you could model this behavior when you eat out or at someone's house; you can remind them when eating at a friend's to say thank you thus providing a little hint that is what you are supposed to do—although I know my kids always say thank you at friends' houses and not always at mine.)

Another way to get them to appreciate the food is to include them in the process. Including them in the process of planning and cooking is helpful for you, and it also makes them realize what you do every day.

As a parent, you don't get a lot of thank you's or pats on the back even if you try to train them to do it. That is one of the reasons that you have to love yourself too, and you have to cut yourself some slack. So when you make a meal plan for the week, and do the shopping and the prep and then there is a wrench thrown into your plans like an unexpected doctor visit or someone having to stay after school longer than expected, or a game running over, and you find yourself having to put aside your plan and punt—don't beat yourself up! Don't get mad because you ended up eating pizza or taking the kids to Chipolte even though you have an amazing dinner either cooked or prepped at home. Go home, figure out if you can repurpose the ingredients from the meal, use it another night or freeze it and move on. You still got to spend the meal with your kids, even if it was in your car or at a restaurant.

Do the best you can and be kind to yourself. Being kind to yourself is something I discuss a lot with my clients. When you are trying to adapt new habits, including eating or lifestyle changes, it can be tough. You have your goals and you know why you are trying to achieve them, but sometimes you misstep, don't make the best choice or go back to an old way. At that time you need to take a breath, acknowledge that it is done, and move on! Maybe you can think a bit about why you did it, how it made you feel, if it was worth it ... but in the end, be kind to yourself and just move on.

Strive for progress not perfection, try to do better but do not have a goal to be perfect. Because no one is perfect. Work on the ADDs and celebrate small successes. If you can get your kids to even think about eating one serving more of fruit of vegetables a day, if you and your kids increase your water daily, if you are doing conscious movement every other day or planning and cooking three meals a week when you used to plan none—celebrate those successes on your journey. Set small attainable goals, baby steps, that you can achieve and feel good about.

One last point on Love... I have encountered a lot of moms who have chosen to stay home with their children who had very successful careers before their kids, or were on their way to successful careers before they decided to stay home, or kept working but not at the same capacity as before kids. For those that did not go back to work or for whom their careers are not what they planned because they have kids, I find that there is sometimes a bit of resentment. Especially if you aren't getting the pats on the backs and the applauds from the audience. I mean who doesn't like a good performance review from your boss, or a raise or bonus! I understand because I feel that way sometimes too, at least I used to.

Give it up! Change your attitude and figure out a way to love it! You know you love your kids and your family, that is why you are doing all of this, and the truth is that retirement from being your kids' primary care giver comes way too quickly! So enjoy it while you can, change your attitude, find some time to do things that you love and enjoy so that you don't feel resentful of having to do the job that you chose—the job of being a parent.

If you are a stay at home parent, realize how blessed you are to be able to do this full time. If you are a working parent, try to put the work behind you when you get home. Be with your kids, love your kids. Remember why you did this. The time we have with our kids while they are young is fleeting, it goes so quickly, so remember to enjoy it and love them and make them feel loved.

OK, enough mushy stuff... let's move on!

• Other Adds •

You cannot turn on the TV these days without hearing about another new superfood that you have to try. You cannot believe everything you hear, and some of the hype is just trying to sell a new product, but Mother Nature is brilliant and has created some foods that do amazing things for our bodies and our health. In trying to keep this book at a basic level, I am not going to go into all of the amazing superfoods that you could ADD. Drinking water, eating more fruits and vegetables, moving, meal planning and Love are a lot for now. But I did want to let you know that when you are ready, there are a ton of amazing foods out there you should try to ADD. A few of my favorites are chia seeds, flax seeds, hemp seeds, cocao, and sea vegetables.

• Self Care •

One last ADD is to schedule time for your own self care. As parents we are so busy and when we do get a chance to breathe, we often do something with or for our kids. Schedule time in your busy schedule (actually make an appointment in your calendar!) to read, take a walk, get a manicure, go on a date with your spouse or significant other, go out with friends, go to a movie or just take a bath!

By taking care of yourself, you are better able to take care of your family. So prioritize this important ADD.

CHAPTER 3
AWARE

We have spent a lot of time discussing the first step ADD. The next step of the ENJOY HEALTHY method is AWARE.

Becoming AWARE of what you are currently doing helps you to see what you are really eating.

• Food Journals •

The first thing I do with my private clients is have them keep a food journal for a few days. This is something that you can do on your own. Just keep track of what you and your family are actually eating. It is always interesting to look at what we really ate versus what we think we ate. When I ask people to do this, I am more concerned with what they are eating and when then with how much. So no need to weigh or measure. Some of my clients just snap pictures on their phones. For some it is helpful to include things such as how they were feeling emotionally and physically before and after they ate to help point out concerns that may need to be addressed like food intolerances or habits that need to be broken.

There are many things you can learn from the exercise of keeping a food journal, both about behavior and the food you are eating.

You may start to realize that you snack at a certain time everyday, even if you are not hungry. You may see that you are eating your own meal and then the kids' left overs or that you eat every night after the kids go to sleep.

Keeping a food journal also helps you become AWARE of what you are eating. You might think that you don't really eat that many processed foods, or that you eat a lot of fruits and vegetables. It isn't until you keep track that you realize that what you think you are doing and what you are actually doing are two different things.

· Pantry Raid & Label Reading ·

Another exercise I do with my private clients is a Pantry Raid. (Not a Panty Raid!) I go to their homes and together we go through their kitchen cabinets and their refrigerator. We look at the food they typically buy, read labels and talk about how they use the food. You can easily do this yourself, but first it is important to know what to look for on a food label.

I know, we learn in school how to read nutritional labels, but I would like to suggest that you start looking at them in a whole different way. Ideally, we wouldn't even have to worry about reading labels because all the food we bought would be single ingredient food that have no labels. Foods like produce, whole grains, fish, meat, etc don't need labels. But I know that is pretty unrealistic for most people including me. So I would just like to have you rethink the way you look at labels and redirect your attention away from the box with numbers and down to the words underneath, that is the ingredients.

When most people look at a nutritional label, they look at the box to see how many calories, carbohydrates, fat, etc. the product has per serving—and they might look at the serving size too. Over the years the government has required companies to put more information in that box to help the consumer be better educated on what they are eating—Thanks! Well, I am here to suggest that you focus more on the ingredients, than the numbers in the box. You can learn all you need to learn about the food you are about to eat or buy by reading that part of the label. (Note: There are some health problems where your doctor may advise you to keep track of things like sodium and grams of sugar. This book is not meant to replace any doctor's recommendation, but even if you are keeping track of a particular number, start looking at ingredients too.)

Reading labels this way will allow you to become AWARE of what you are really eating. So here are my guidelines for label reading and what to look for in the ingredients.

1. You should be able to read all the ingredients listed and have a pretty good idea of what each of the ingredients is. (If it has high fructose corn syrup or hydrogenated oils, put it back.)

2. The fewer the ingredients the better.

3. Ideally you want food that could pass a kitchen test, that is, could someone with a reasonable amount of skill in the kitchen make this from scratch? Are there chemicals or ingredients that you can't buy as single ingredients at the grocery store? Are there ingredients that are highly processed like white flour, white rice, white sugar or starches where many of the nutrients have been stripped away?

These guidelines above are in order of importance, so I would not expect every item in your pantry to be able to pass the "kitchen test." But by following these guidelines you will become AWARE of how much processed food you are eating and what is really in your food!

The ingredients that you cannot read, or do not know what they are, or sound like they were made in a laboratory should be avoided. There are so many that I am not going to go into each one, but some of them are really bad for you and many of them were created to trick your body into eating more of the food (scary!), so my general rule is to try to stay away the best I can!

Choose foods where the whole ingredient is intact, like whole wheat flour, and brown rice, instead of their nutrient stripped counterparts.

I have participated in a challenge to try to avoid processed foods for a month. I have done it and it is harder than you think, but talk about becoming AWARE of how much processed foods you eat!

Yes, reading labels does take time and I vowed to help save you time, but I also want you to eat real, healthy food. The most healthy ingredients don't have labels to read (produce like apples, carrots and kale, grains like quinoa or rice, fish, meat...). Also, this is a one-time thing. Yes, you will now be reading labels more closely, but you do not have to read a label every time you purchase a food. If during your pantry raid, you find an item that does not meet the guidelines, next time you go to the store to replenish it, you will have to read labels to ADJUST, and find a good substitute but this is a one time thing. Once you have done your research, you don't need to recheck every time. (Although with the way the food manufacturers change ingredients on us, it is not a bad idea to spot check every so often.)

Now you know how to read a food label, looking for good ingredients instead of just at the numbers. This will help you make better choices and avoid marketing traps. I used to be in marketing. I was a product manager whose job it was to make my product more appealing to the consumer and get them to buy more! So I know how these people work. They tell you what you want to hear and trust me they know what you want to hear because they have done a lot of research to figure it out. But now you are smarter than them! If a product says "all natural" or has some health claim, yet still contains a lot of ingredients you cannot read and were obviously made in a plant not grown on a plant, you know to put it back on the shelf! They can't fool you anymore.

My clients are often shocked when they become AWARE of what they are actually eating in all those processed foods.

· Home Cooking ·

A food journal and pantry raid can open your eyes not just to what is in the food you are eating, but how much processed/ prepared or convenience foods you actually eat. I am always amazed when I ask my clients how much they cook at home. For most people, it is a lot less than I would expect it to be. Busy families end up "picking something up" a lot! Then for those that say they cook at home, it turns out that they are not really cooking, but reheating store bought, frozen, or processed foods.

I challenge you to ask yourself: How much food you use in your "cooking" is made in a plant and doesn't come from a plant? Or is from the center aisles of the grocery store? How often do you pick something up for dinner? How often do you "cook" a frozen dinner? How often does your family eat out?

When we talk about home cooking, once again the hurdle of time is encountered. It is time consuming to cook your meals, from scratch. There is a reason why the center of the grocery store where all the processed/convenience foods are has grown so much over the past decades; people are spending more time and money there than in the outer portions of the store where the fresh foods are located.

Most people do not really think about how much of their food someone else made. Having food that reduces the amount of time we spend in the kitchen is very appealing, but there are also sacrifices, usually to the quality of ingredients and often to our health. Through the pantry raid and food journal, you will become AWARE of how much processed food you may be eating. Highly processed foods cause all types of health issues that may not manifest themselves at the time we eat them but can cause issues over time, or are causing problems in our bodies that we don't even know about.

You may be thinking, the title of this book talks about saving time. How can I save time if I am cooking everything from scratch? Well, I will give you some great tips for saving time, and making this whole process easier, and less time consuming. Right now I don't want you to think about the extra time it will take (or not take), I just want you to become AWARE of what and how much you are cooking and think about how you can ADD more home cooked meals to your family's routine.

· Sugar, Soy, Dairy and Wheat, Oh My! ·

Every day we see a new article or news story about some food which we should or should not be eating. Sugar, Soy, Dairy and Wheat (Gluten) are hot topics right now, and I get a lot of questions/ comments about them from my clients. As with most foods, my opinion is usually if you have diversity in your diet, and aren't always eating the same things, you will probably be OK. (There are some exceptions like allergies and intolerances of course.) The thing is that most people don't realize how much of a certain food they eat because they are eating processed foods that sneak stuff in without us knowing.

My goal is not to tell you to restrict or eliminate these or other ingredients, but for you to become AWARE of how much you are eating.

Often times I hear from clients, "Sugar really isn't an issue, I don't eat a lot of sweets" or "I don't need to worry about soy since I don't eat tofu" or "I don't really drink milk or eat cheese, I just use a little milk in my coffee" or "I feel fine when I eat gluten or wheat and I actually don't really eat that much." Then we start reading labels....

The good news is that with new labeling, milk, soy and wheat are listed as allergens and therefore easy to find if we just look at the end of the ingredients list. Sugar is a little more difficult as it goes by many names and is in places you would never expect it.

Here is a list of just some (50) of the names sugar goes by:

* Barley malt
* Beet sugar
* Brown sugar
* Buttered syrup
* Cane juice crystals
* Cane sugar
* Caramel
* Corn syrup
* Corn syrup solids
* Confectioner's sugar
* Carob syrup
* Castor sugar
* Date sugar
* Demerara sugar
* Dextran
* Dextrose
* Diastatic malt
* Diatase
* Ethyl maltol
* Fructose
* Fruit juice
* Fruit juice concentrate
* Galactose
* Glucose
* Glucose solids
* Golden sugar
* Golden syrup
* Grape sugar
* High-fructose corn syrup
* Honey
* Icing sugar
* Invert sugar
* Lactose
* Maltodextrin
* Maltose
* Malt syrup
* Maple syrup
* Molasses
* Muscovado sugar
* Panocha
* Raw sugar
* Refiner's syrup
* Rice syrup
* Sorbitol
* Sorghum syrup
* Sucrose
* Sugar
* Treacle
* Turbinado sugar
* Yellow sugar

So if you are one of those people who think that they don't eat a lot of sugar, start checking your labels. You may be surprised to see that sugar is hiding in your bread, and in your pasta sauce!

Although natural sugars like maple syrup and honey and sugar in fruits and even vegetables are better for you than refined sugars, they are still sugar. There is so much information out there now about what effects sugar is having on our bodies. My take-away from all of this information is that sugar, especially refined sugar, is what is making us fat and causing a lot of diseases; sugar makes us hungrier, and we eat a lot more sugar than we think we do!

This is the same with soy, dairy and wheat. My main concern with soy is that most of the soy we eat is highly processed and often genetically modified. If you "don't eat tofu," once you start checking labels you will become AWARE of how much soy you are actually eating! Soy is an ingredient in a lot of processed foods, places you would never even imagine. I am not saying you should never eat it, but wouldn't you like to know when you are and have it be your choice?

My goal in this book is to help you and your family eat more real, whole foods and make lifestyle changes to support you in achieving your goal of feeding your family healthy meals with less stress, money and time. My goal is not to preach about dairy and gluten and why they are or are not bad for you. So I will keep my comments on them brief.

There is a lot of research and information out there about why you may want to avoid dairy and gluten (the protein found in wheat and some other grains). Everything from people having unknown allergies and intolerances, to them triggering autoimmune diseases, to them being the cause of your stiffness, stuffy nose or break outs. Personally I feel better not eating them.

When I do cleanses or detoxes with people, I ask them to eliminate these items as well as soy and some other things for the short time of the detox. After, we add them back in one at a time to determine if there is a reaction or sensitivity. This is what is referred to as an elimination diet and it is a good way to determine if you have an issue with a food. Often people will be very surprised at the results. People who tell me that dairy isn't an issue will realize that they get bloating and gassy or become very congested or break out after reintroducing it. The same with gluten, maybe it is that they become lethargic or have stomach pains after. For some with autoimmune diseases, they have found that by eliminating dairy and/or gluten they have been able to reverse the symptoms of their disease.

Again, this book is not about food sensitivities and allergies, or about how to go gluten or dairy free (although I have lots of ideas on that), whether or not you decide to try to test your sensitivity, my goal if for you to become AWARE of what you are eating.

That is what AWARE is all about! Being AWARE of what we are actually eating versus what we think we are eating. Once we are AWARE, we are more in control and can decide to ADJUST.

CHAPTER 4

ADJUST

We've covered a lot of information in a short time. You know what to ADD, and you know to become AWARE. The next step then is to ADJUST your current habits and behavior.

Now that we are AWARE, it is time to determine where you can ADJUST.

ADJUST is different than ADD because ADD is where we adopt new habits or incorporate new items and ADJUST is where we make changes to what we are already doing. Some ADDs may actual turn out to be ADJUSTs. Like when you ADD leafy greens to your dinner plate and it decreases the amount of animal protein you eat—that is an ADJUST without even trying.

With both ADD and ADJUST it is important to set realistic goals that you can easily obtain, so you will be motivated to keep going. Such as, ADD one green vegetable a day or make a home made dinner twice a week.

· Upgrade Your Ingredients ·

Now that you are reading labels, and are AWARE of what is really in all of the processed food you are eating, you can ADJUST and find better alternatives.

Of course the biggest ADJUST should be to eat less processed foods and more real whole foods, so label reading would become less of an issue. For the foods you do buy pre-made, read your labels and determine if maybe you need to ADJUST the brand you buy. If your jar of spaghetti sauce has sugar in it, find one that doesn't or start making your own. If your juice has high fructose corn syrup, look for 100% juice, and read the label to make sure that all that is in there is juice. If you worry that it might be more expensive, water it down, or better yet, drink less.

By upgrading your ingredients and filling your pantry and refrigerator with good stuff, you take a major step in the right direction.

This works in recipes too! If you have a recipe you love, see if you can ADJUST the ingredients. Maybe you can add in more vegetables or change the type of oil/fat that is used. Being healthy does not mean giving up everything you love to eat. Deprivation is not enjoyable! Now that you are AWARE, you can make some changes that may allow you to have a delicious new healthier version, just by swapping some ingredients or using a different technique.

I will talk more about this idea of upgrading ingredients and doing recipe makeovers a little later. Finding things your family wants to eat is usually challenging enough, we don't want to mess with it too much and then have them tell us they don't want to eat it!

· Plate ·

Another thing you can ADJUST is the composition of your plate, or the way that you think about your meals.

Some people get a little worried when I start talking about eating "mainly plants." Although being vegan or vegetarian is a good option for some, for others it might not be best for their health or they just might not want to stop eating meat! That is fine!

ADJUST the way you plan your meals. Instead of thinking of the animal protein like chicken, beef or pork as being the star of the show, have it be a supporting character and a really high quality-supporting actor. I use this analogy because we have all seen shows or movies where the supporting character steals the show or is an important part of the storyline. Just because meat has less real estate on the plate doesn't mean it cannot be an impactful part of the meal.

I challenge you to make the stars—the veggies and the grains — amazing too! Watching a boring moving with horrible acting just for the supporting actor isn't really that enjoyable. We want the movie to be fabulous and then have the bonus of the supporting actor sending it over the top! (Do you like the way I got something about movies in here? Creating a meal is like producing a movie—I keep trying!)

· Grass-Fed, Wild, Organic Meat and Fish ·

When I start talking about upgrading ingredients,many of my clients start to ask about words like Grass Fed and Organic.

Animal products are one place it is truly important to upgrade your ingredients. And since we are eating less quantity wise, we can afford to increase the quality. Like us, if an animal is fed poor quality food, or genetically modified food or food that it was not meant to eat, it can affect the health and the composition of the animal. When we eat that animal, those "defects" are passed on to us.

For example, cows were made to eat grass. Ideally all cows would all be "happy cows" as my nephew calls them and they would spend their days grazing in a pasture on healthy untreated grass, until the time when they were humanely taken for their meat. The anatomy of a cow is made for it to eat grass; when cows eat other things like corn, it causes the meat of the animal to be more marbled, which tastes great, but is means more saturated fat. It also has less Omega 3's and more Omega 6's which have been shown to cause inflammation. But let's keep it simple.

You should buy the best quality animal products you can afford. Remembering what the animal was fed and how it was treated during its life does affect the meat that you are eating.

This also applies to fish. We hear that fish is good for us, but again where it was raised, and what it was fed impacts the health benefits of the fish. We want to mainly eat fish that has more of the good stuff, like Omega 3's, and less of the bad stuff, like mercury. The Environmental Working Group (ewg.org) has a seafood guide and I find it is a good reference to help determine what type of fish from where I should be choosing at the store.

· Organics—everything else! ·

We see this word everywhere now! But does it mean it is always better and do we need to buy everything organic? There is a lot of research supporting the idea that eating organic is better for us and it is definitely better for the environment. But again this is an area where you have to make the right decisions for you and your family and do a little research on your own.

Organics are usually more expensive than their "conventional" counterparts. I know that this impacts many people's decision whether or not to buy organic. My advice is to do a little research and make decisions that are best for your family given what is available, and what fits in your budget.

The Environmental Working group (ewg.org) again is a great resource to help with your decisions about organics. The Dirty Dozen and Clean Fourteen are lists they put together annually to help determine which produce you should prioritize buying organic when available. I use these lists to help guide me with my choices. Also, if it is produce where I am going to eat the skin or the part of the plant that is exposed to a potential pesticide I try to choose organic. Particularly items like berries, apples and greens, although I try to buy organic whenever it is available and not cost prohibitive! This concept also influences my decision when buying items (or even making home made) like fresh juice, applesauce or baby food, as not only are the skins usually included, but it is a concentrated amount of the item so I will usually choose organic. Items like citrus, bananas and avocados that have a thick skin, I usually do not buy organic, given that I peel them and rarely eat the skin (except maybe for the occasional zesting).

I also get the impression that not all organics are created equal! I would rather buy from a smaller local, responsible farmer who maybe just hasn't gone for the Organic Certification than from a larger company where the organic produce has had to travel a great distance to get to me. My favorite is the organic booths at the farmers markets—local and organic! Or you can join an organic CSA (Community Supported Agriculture). With a CSA, not only do you know where your food is coming from, but it can actually help with meal planning and new produce experimentation. Many CSAs are now sending out the list of the weekly share contents before delivery with recipes. Often there is produce in the box that is not in your normal repertoire, so it forces you to be adventurous and try something new!

As for items that are not in the produce aisle, I will often choose organic to help ensure I am not buying GMOs (Genetically Modified Organisms—meaning they have done something in the lab to alter the organism; for example, making a bug resistant crop of corn.) Until GMO labeling on all foods is mandatory (keeping fingers crossed), it is hard to know how the ingredients listed were grown. Buying organic should mean buying non-GMO. As I mentioned before with things like soy so prevalent in the ingredient lists on our food, knowing that it is non-GMO helps. Also, if I am buying something like pasta sauce or vegetable broth (no, I don't always make my own—I am a busy mom remember), I want to make sure that the vegetables going in are the same as I would use if I were to make it myself.

With organics in higher demand, they are becoming easier to find. The wholesale clubs are caring more organic items, and there are now a lot of sources online. Although I like to stick to my local market or farmers market for my fresh produce, I will buy pantry items like quinoa, rice, or chia seeds in bulk at Costco. I don't recommend doing this to try new items. For that I recommend the bulk bins at the grocery store so you can buy a smaller amount to try, but once you know that you will use two pounds of quinoa before it goes bad—go for it! Another place to look is in the frozen foods aisle. I buy large bags of organic frozen berries for our smoothies, and there are always bags or organic frozen veggies in my freezer. Frozen is often more economical, and is usually frozen close to time it is picked, so many nutrients are well preserved.

One word of caution on organics… just because a product is organic, doesn't mean it is "healthy." All the reading label rules still apply!

My goal in this book is to help you on your journey to feeding your family healthy meals. Everyone who picks up this book is at a different point in her journey, and I don't want to overwhelm people just starting. When you are ready, do a little of your own research on grass fed, organic, wild, etc. and figure out what will work best for you and your family.

· Behaviors ·

When you do your food journal, you might become AWARE of some behaviors as they relate to food. Like snacking a lot, eating off of your kid's plate, eating when you are bored or eating late at night.

Although these behaviors are not necessarily bad, once you become AWARE of them, it leads you to be able to ADJUST them if necessary. Maybe you realize you don't need that snack or you change what it is you are snacking on. Since you are now AWARE that you are picking at your kids' leftovers, you can ADJUST and eat with them so you are not hungry or you just stop eating them. At night, you ADJUST to just have a cup of tea instead of food once they go to sleep. How you ADJUST your behavior depends on your health goals.

Notice your family's behaviors and rhythms as well. Are your kids eating a snack right before dinner, so they are not hungry at meal time? Are they hungry after dinner? Becoming AWARE can help you ADJUST. Maybe you have dinner earlier, or give them more of a meal at snack time and then a lighter dinner. Review what you are eating at dinner - do you need to bulk it up or make some changes so that they won't be coming back hungry later? Maybe it is a habit to eat again while doing homework (or even a procrastination tool). Perhaps instead of eating, you can point out another way for your kids to take a break like using the time to shower, call a friend, jam out on an instrument, shoot a few hoops or dance to their favorite song (just remind them to keep track of the time). If they really are hungry, offer a healthy snack.

Thinking through a list of alternatives to eating when not hungry is a great idea for anyone for whom this is an issue. Now that you are aware of what you are doing, you can catch yourself and go to your "list." Maybe go for a walk, or drink some water, or go to another room in the house when you feel the urge to eat when not hungry.

As you can see, ADJUST does not have to be overwhelming. Making small changes will have a big impact.

CHAPTER 5
ENJOY

The last step actually takes no work at all. Once you ADD in the good stuff, become AWARE of what you are currently doing and ADJUST where necessary, ENJOY just comes naturally.

You will ENJOY knowing that you are feeding your family healthy foods, ENJOY not having the looming question of "what's for dinner" over you head every day, ENJOY achieving your and your families health goals, ENJOY having more time to spend doing things you want to do, ENJOY less stress, ENJOY looking and feeling great, and maybe even ENJOY your job as Mom more than you already do!

The Concepts of **ADD, AWARE, ADJUST, ENJOY**™ are not complicated, but they do take a little getting used to and a little up front work. Now let's look at some tools you can use to help implement this strategy in your home. This is when you can really begin to ENJOY HEALTHY!

PART 2: THE TOOLKIT

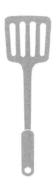

CHAPTER 6
BUILDING YOUR TEAM

Building your arsenal of recipes to feed your family is a lot like building a team. You have your star fan favorites who you know will play well and everyone will love watching (or eating, in this case); you have your back up players who are reliable and there when you need them but don't really get that much attention from the crowd; and you have your back up players you just brought up from the minor leagues who you need to try out to see how they will work. And as we know, some days even the star players don't play as well as expected, or the fans aren't as happy as they usually are with their performance.

• Fan favorites •

We all know how it is; we plan, prep and cook a meal and then when it gets to the table, it gets a not so fabulous response from the fans—i.e. our family. To help solve this problem, it is important to get your family involved in the process. That is why the first step in my meal planning process is to create a family favorites list.

This is an easy exercise (in theory; yes, I have teenagers too). Each family members needs to come up with at least 3 Breakfasts, 3 lunches, 3 dinners, 3 sides and 3 snacks that they like and will eat—no questions asked. (Later when I talk about weekly planning, the concept of asking them what they want that week will come up, but for now this is just a go-to list).

I've included a worksheet for you to use for this process. (Note: All of the worksheets in this book are in the Appendix, as well as available for you to download on my website at www.enjoyhealthy.me)

Family Food List

Breakfast	Lunch	Dinner	Sides	Snacks

Notes

© 2015 *If I Could Just Cook In My Car* • enjoyhealthy.me

Family Food List

If your kids don't want to contribute to the list then they don't get a say, and they just eat what is put in front of them. In my house, especially when my kids were little, there was always the "other option." If you didn't like what I was serving, there was always yogurt or PB&J that you could get for yourself. Now my kids can make themselves eggs or soup or something, because I am only cooking once.

Having this go-to list will help when doing your weekly meal plan. You can categorize the list by prep time, method of cooking (like slow cooker), being able to make in advance, and even give it a grade as to how much you and your family like it. You don't really have to "categorize it" unless you are that organized—which I am not, but it is good to review the list and the recipes whether written or not, that go with the meal to help you determine how they will fit in to your weekly plan. I recommend you do this with all your recipes.

Speaking of recipes, once you have your list, it is a good time to review the recipes to determine if any of them need a "makeover." Using **ADD, AWARE, ADJUST, ENJOY**™ concepts, you can review the recipe and become AWARE of any ADDS or ADJUSTS you may want to make. Maybe you can ADD more veggies, or ADJUST the breadcrumbs and use whole wheat instead of white.

This is a dynamic list; you can grow or change it as often as you want or need. Maybe after a few tries, your child remembers he doesn't really like one of the items he put on the list. Take it off. And of course when you find a new recipe or idea that you LOVE, add it to the list!

One thing you might have noticed missing on the family favorite list is dessert. Some families have dessert every night, some just on occasion. I am not anti-dessert, it is personally my favorite part of the meal, but in our house it not a planned part of the meal. If someone wants something for dessert there is always fruit, usually sorbetto and maybe some homemade cookies (or store bought on occasion). Typical desserts usually have a lot of refined sugar, refined flour, "bad' oils and a lot of other stuff that may not be the best for you. Make sure to read the label and check. Homemade desserts where you control the ingredients are a much better choice and there are tons of them out there. If you want to add dessert to your family favorite list so that you have some on hand, great! You just might have to ADJUST some of the options or maybe just have them on occasion.

· Back Up Players ·

You should also contribute your favorites to this list, but you can also add the things that maybe others may have forgotten. Those old faithful meals that no one is running home for, but everyone will eat. Also, consider things like Garbage Soup and Garbage Salad (when you just make soup or salad from what you have on hand). Freezer meals can go on this list if your family hasn't already added them. Maybe they like stuffed shells from a favorite restaurant or Costco; just remember to review ingredients to become AWARE of what is really in there. You can always try another brand or use it as an occasional easy prep dinner.

On our list, I put things like French Bread Pizza. Whenever we have leftover baguettes from a meal or I buy individual baguettes in bulk, I slice and freeze the extra. When my kids need a quick dinner, I take out the bread, pop it in the microwave for 30 seconds or so, then in the toaster, add sauce, cheese, and toppings (including lots of veggies—broccoli and olives are my family favorite) and put it back in the toaster. I put out some lettuce and dressings and have a quick meal for the kids.

Along these lines you should have some "pantry" meals as well. Pasta, quinoa, canned beans and jarred sauces all can be used for a quick meal, especially when you have your freezer stocked with some frozen vegetables that you can add. Although we don't make pasta as a main meal a lot, once in a while I will make pasta (plain or gluten free), open up a jar of sauce and "doctor it up" with frozen veggies like broccoli or spinach and maybe some olives. Easy, quick, delicious and filling!

Since you have stocked your pantry with pasta and sauce that have good ingredients, you can feel good about this quick meal. I also have Ramen noodles—of course they are "healthy" ones with approved ingredients — on hand in my pantry. My daughter actually cooks the noodles and then puts vegan bouillon in instead of the included spices or she makes rice vermicelli noodles and adds them to bouillon she has made as the broth. Toss in a few mushrooms or frozen veggies and you have a healthy snack. I have included the Sanderson Family list as an example and some of our favorite recipes are in the back. (This was my daughter Paige's idea—you can thank her!)

Sanderson Family Food List

Breakfast	Lunch	Dinner	Sides/Snacks
Nutella® with strawberries or Bananas	Wraps - Chicken or Turkey	Stuffed Shells	Kale chips
Eggs	PB&J	Chili	Salad
PB&J	Soup	Burgers	Mashed potatoes
Toast	Peanut Butter with apple and Pretzels	Chicken/eggplant "Parm"	Sweet potato chips
Waffles	Hummus and Veggies	Roast Chicken	Whole sweet potatoes
Pancakes	Fried Rice	Quesadillas	Veggies- roasted, steamed
Smoothies	Pasta Salad	Fajitas/tacos - veggie, meat, fish	Spinach and mushrooms sautéed
Granola and yogurt	Chicken nuggets	Thai lettuce wraps	Quinoa with veggies
Toast with avocado	Salad	Spring rolls	"Fries"
Cereal	Pasta	Mussels	Popcorn - maple, smart pop
Oatmeal - overnight or instant	Rice with cucumber and avocado	Fish: pan seared/in parchment	Hummus and veggies
Fruit		Grilled veggie sandwiches	Guacamole with veggies
		Chicken Cesar salad with garlic pita	Nachos with guacamole and salsa
		Potato Bar	Corn on the cob
		Turkey/veggie chili	
		Pulled chicken	
		Pizza breads	
		Shepard's pie	
		Hot dogs and/or hamburgers	
		Buffalo broc/cauliflower and wings	
		Zucchini pasta with pesto or other sauce	
		Pasta with Alfredo or veggie sauce	
		Turkey meatball subs	

Notes

© 2015 *If I Could Just Cook In My Car* • enjoyhealthy.me

Sanderson Family Food List Example

• Adding to your Roster •

This can be the fun part, but also the overwhelming part especially when it comes to new recipes. Cooking School 101 —when you get a new recipe, make sure to read through the whole thing! There might be a technique that you don't know how to do, or prep that needs to be done hours or days before. Also, there may be ingredients that are new to you. The worst is when you have to buy an expensive, unique ingredient for that amazing new recipe only to find out that you don't like the recipe and you will never use the rest of that ingredient (usually a spice for me). In that situation I do one of two things. I either skip the recipe or I try to substitute for the ingredients or modify the recipe. Yummy, healthy food does not have to be difficult. If the recipe looks over complicated or has a ton of new ingredients, skip it!

There are many ways to add to your roster including childhood favorites, friends, internet searches, blogs, magazines, cookbooks and restaurant menus.

Childhood Favorites

Think back to when you were a kid, what did you eat? More importantly, what did you like to eat? You might need to find a better alternative to the Hungry Man dinner that you looked forward to when your parents went out for the night and you got to eat it out of that metal tray in front of the TV. (I loved those nights, the mashed potatoes, meatloaf and most importantly the cobbler—YUM!)

Your childhood favorites can easily become your family favorites. You might not even have to do that much "work" to the recipe. My mom wasn't the most gourmet cook (sorry, Mom) and she never really used spices (outside of Lawry's Season Salt) or things like onions or garlic and many ingredients she used then we now know aren't the best for us because they contain things like MSG or hydrogenated oil, but those are easy fixes.

Mom used to make these yummy sweet and sour meatballs. When I was first married we used to have a holiday party with all of our friends and I always made the sweet and sour meatballs. Over time, it got harder to have an adult party at that crazy time of year, so we switched to family friendly Christmas in July parties where the food switched from adult hors d'oeuvres to kid friendly BBQ.

I forgot about those meatballs, until someone asked for the recipe. The recipe is super easy. Take one jar of grape jelly and one jar of chili sauce and dump them in a pot. Turn on heat and let them "melt" together and then add ground beef rolled into balls to the liquid, cover and cook until done, serve with mini rye bread. I know it may sound gross, but they are amazing! Once reminded of how much I love these things—and who wouldn't, they are pretty much meat covered in sugar - I decided to make them for my family.

I bought grass fed ground beef, and found grape jelly and chili sauce that was organic without high fructose corn syrup or anything else I couldn't read. (By the way, if you try to make these—this is the chili sauce that looks like cocktail sauce, usually with the BBQ sauce and ketchup, not the Asian one, but that could be good too!) I also made some vegan meatballs for myself, but used the same sauce. Oh the memories! I steamed some broccoli and served the broccoli and meatballs over brown rice—YUM! Truth is my family actually did not like them as much as I did—they said they were too sweet!

I tell you this story to show that recipes are easily trans-formed or "upgraded" by changing a few ingredients. For my mom's "lemon chicken," she breaded chicken with egg and seasoned breadcrumbs then pan fried it slightly, put it in a baking pan and covered it with liquid she had made using water, a bunch of bouillon cubes and some good squirts of the lemon juice that came out of the plastic lemon. Then she added canned sliced mushrooms and cooked in the oven until done. (This is how Mom cooked—no recipes, just do this, then this, then done. I actually love cooking like that.)

This lemon chicken is probably one of my kid's favorites from Grandma. They've been eating it since they could eat solid food. So of course I copied it, but again I used different whole-wheat breadcrumbs and bouillon that didn't have MSG or hydrogenated oils. I used chicken broth as the liquid, adding a few vegan bouil-lon cubes for flavor and fresh lemon juice. Fresh mushrooms (sautéed first to give them the right consistency) are substituted for canned which had some extra ingredients I didn't like. I still fried it before I cooked it (but in olive oil instead of canola), so the texture was the same.

As you can see, recipe makeovers don't have to be difficult. Although my family eats differently than I did as a kid, with lighter meals more focused on veggies, you can get inspiration from what you loved as a kid.

Friends

Friends are a great resource for meal ideas. I constantly ask my friends what they feed their families. People are also sharing recipes today on social media—like Facebook and Pinterest. People seem to love to take pictures of their food and share it, especially if they made something impressive and delicious!

You could start a recipe-sharing group with some friends, like a book club (gives you an excuse to get together and drink wine.) You can even share your weekly meal plans, and even better, maybe get a group together and share the cooking. Everyone makes a big batch of one thing and shares it with the others. If you have friends or live in a community where that would work, try it!

Internet/Blogs

As I mentioned before, we are lucky to have at our fingertips access to unlimited information (although there are negatives to this as well, but not going there now). There are so many recipes on the internet that you could never have to use the same recipe twice. If you have an ingredient on hand that you want to use, just search for recipes with that ingredient. If there is a type of food you like, search it and find a recipe. I find that I use the internet more for when I have something on hand that I want to use, or if I have an idea, but not a plan.

For example, one night I had planned to make tacos. I realized that I did not have a packet of taco seasoning, probably because I couldn't find one where I liked the ingredients. I searched for homemade taco seasoning and looked through a few recipes until I found one that looked good and for which I had all the ingredients on hand. I think I might have even combined a few recipes. A quick search saved me and kept our dinner on track.

The internet is also a resource when you need to find a substitution for an ingredient you don't have or don't want to "invest" in for one dish. As we know, people post everything so you can also find videos to help you with any cooking technique or to find any information on how to handle or prepare an unfamiliar food item.

During your searches you are bound to find some sites that you really like, especially if you are doing specific searches. I often search for vegan options or dairy and/or gluten free. You might search for broccoli recipes for picky eaters. When you find a site that appeals to you, first book mark it so that it can be a go-to for you, and then look to see if they have a mailing list. I know our inboxes are really full, but subscribing to a few sites that appeal to you could be very helpful. Signing up can put interesting blogs with new recipes in your inbox on a regular basis. Subscribers to my list not only get my blog post delivered directly to their inbox, but also get a weekly menu (usually what my family is eating that week) with links to all the recipes on my website.

Most people with websites also have a social media presence, so you can "like" them on Facebook or view them on Pinterest to provide a stream of new ideas.

Media

With the popularity of cooking shows, you can turn on the TV any time of day and find some cooking show. Once you find one that you like and whose tastes are similar to yours, you can learn a lot by watching a few of them. More likely than not they also have a web page where you can get their recipes.

These shows are a great way to get the kids involved and inspired. My kids and I watch shows like *Chopped* and *Cuthroat Kitchen* on the Food Network or any of the other "challenges" shows. Not only has it inspired my daughter to want to be a chef and for both of my girls to want to get into the kitchen more, but sometimes it inspires our meals: This is what we have on hand, what can we make, or that looks so delicious, let's try to make that.

There are also cooking segments on many other shows, like morning talk shows. Sometimes there are good ideas or interesting recipes and most often they are quick and easy—you have to be able to show it in a short segment so even though their prep is done for them before, the recipe still needs to be relatively quick. After the segment airs, you can check out the show's website for that recipe and archived recipes too.

I know there is a lot of free stuff on the internet, but let's not forget magazines. I have a few food/cooking magazines to which I subscribe. I often look at the magazines at the check out counter and every so often I will buy one, and then if I really like it I will subscribe either electronically or get the physical magazine. Again, most of their recipes are on the website so even if I stop getting the magazine I might visit the website as a resource. I also enjoy the other content, and learn a lot about food from these sources.

Cookbooks

Personally I LOVE cookbooks! I usually only use one or two recipes from each, but I love having them and looking through them. Once you find someone that you like and start following them, you might want to get their cookbook. When I get a new cookbook, I look through and tag all the recipes I want to try, but I also use cookbooks as a resource when I am searching for a particular recipe—like oatmeal chocolate chip cookies or a nut ball or bar.

Most recipes are now online, so cookbooks like regular books probably aren't as popular, but often cookbooks will provide more than just the recipes. I find that especially "healthy" cookbooks provide background on the ingredients, methods and overall healthy eating guidelines, which can be very informative, and a useful resource.

Restaurant Menus

One last place where I like to get inspired for my meal planning is restaurants. When we go out and my kids really like something they had, I will often try to re-create it at home. I often use the internet to help figure it out. We were at the Cheesecake Factory and my kids were eating Thai Lettuce wraps, which they really enjoy and always do when we go there. Lightbulb! Why don't I just make those at home? I searched for Cheesecake Factory Thai Lettuce Wrap Recipe and got a bunch of options with posts that included the recipes for every part including the dipping sauces. I have played with it a bit, substituting some ingredients and such, and admit I use store bought sauces, but it is now a family favorite. (and my recipe is included with the recipes in the back of the book.)

No matter where you get the ideas from, it is important to be able to have access to them when you need them. There are many ways to organize recipes both in hard copy form and digitally. Maybe you like to have hard copies, so you print every recipe or take it from a magazine and file in a notebook. Or you might be more tech savvy and have all your recipes "pinned" to your Pinterest page. Whatever works for you, just so that when you want to include that player on the roster, you can find them in the dugout!

As you can see, you will never run out of ways to find recipe ideas!

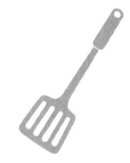

CHAPTER 7

YOUR TOOLS

This book is a guide to save you time, money and stress. By implementing the ADD, AWARE and ADJUST steps, you can ENJOY HEALTHY in your busy life! I hope you can see that it is not that difficult, it just takes a little time to start thinking in this new way. There are "tools" to helps. One investment for your kitchen can save you time, money and stress:.the slow cooker. And don't forget that other all-important and overlooked wonder, the freezer.

• Slow Cooker •
and Other Time Saving Ideas

Slow Cooker

My mother never used a slow cooker, so this was a new concept for me. My first Crock Pot was handed down to me by someone, and the only time I used it was to keep my sweet and sour meatballs hot at my holiday party. A few years ago I asked for a new slow cooker for the holidays. The first thing I cooked in my brand new slow cooker was brisket for Hanukkah! Ironic, given that I don't eat meat and I planned to use this wonderful new device to cook beans and grains and other amazing vegan/vegetarian items that needed a lot of time to cook.

Since then I have found this device is a busy mom's best friend. You know those nights, when you are not really sure when anyone is going to eat, let alone when you are going to cook, because you have back to back to back drop offs and pick ups from different activities and events? (The nights that really inspired the title of this book.) Or maybe you are just running around from the time school ends until dinner time, or your kids' schedules are crazy and they all need dinner at different times or if you work outside the home and just get home from work at dinner time, those are all times when the slow cooker is a savior!

For most recipes, you dump the ingredients in the slow cooker and turn it on—hours later, it is done. A hot meal is ready when family members need it or when you all get home (and bonus, the house smells great!). I recommend investing in a decent slow cooker. I like mine because I can use the insert on the stove so no extra pots to clean. You can also get one with a delay timer so you can set it to start at a later time. Slow cooker recipes abound and you can experiment on how to cook some family favorites in the slow cooker. Honestly, it can be as easy as dumping in some chicken with some sauce and setting the timer.

My family's favorite slow cooker meals are beef stew and pulled chicken. The stew has a bit more prep since I put a lot of veggies in it. What I do is prep the veggies the night before, then in the morning I quickly brown the beef (which you don't really need to do, I just do) and then dump everything in, and set the timer. At dinner time, I quickly make some mashed potatoes (from a box, just check those ingredients!) and serve the stew on top. Serving it this way I avoid having to do the roux (flour and water) to thicken the stew, the mashed potatoes does the job. For the pulled chicken, I just put the chicken and the sauce ingredients (which sometimes I pre-measure the night before) in the pot and turn it on. Some yummy rolls to make sandwiches, or rice to make bowls, and a green salad and dinner is done.

My main reason for using a slow cooker is convenience. It is often quick prep and you can cook while you are not at home without leaving your oven on. For example, I reheat frozen stuffed shells in the slow cooker. Before I go pick up the kids, I dump the shells and the sauce in the cooker, and let it cook it for a few hours. This is a great meal for those nights when everyone is eating at different times. When they need to eat, they go over and get some shells.

Of course another benefit of slow cooking is that cooking things at low heat for an extended period of time often adds to the flavor and texture of the recipe. Meat cooked in the slow cooker is always tender (as long as you have enough liquid—yup, you only make that mistake once) and stews and soup's flavors are more complex when they have the opportunity to cook longer. The slow cooker is like leaving items on simmer for an extended period without having to worry about the stove top being on. If you want to venture into cooking things that take a long time like beans or stocks, the slow cooker is a great tool. Again, you can leave the ingredients cooking for a long time without having to worry about the stove and without having to be home.

I want to mention another great device—the rice cooker. I admit I cannot cook rice, not sure why, but it never works. So I got a rice cooker to solve that problem. It also helps me out because of that fancy delay cooking timer and because it can cook while I am not home. Rice takes a while to cook so being able to come home to a pot of warm rice to use for a meal is a time saver. I often make extra so that there are leftovers to use for another recipe like my "fried rice" or to use in a rice bowl with whatever is in the fridge for lunch. As a note, you do want to soak the rice before you cook it, so it does take a little pre-planning. Soak it overnight if possible and then rinse very well before cooking. If you forget to soak, just make sure to rinse really well. Most rice cookers also work as steamers so again you can set a timer and have steamed veggies ready when you get home.

Invest in a slow cooker and/or rice cooker so that you can actually cook while in your car!

Freezer

The freezer can definitely be a savior when in a pinch or when you forget something at the store and need a quick substitute. I keep mine stocked with lots of frozen veggies, fruits, soups, meat and easy meals. I don't have a huge refrigerator in my kitchen, but I do have an extra refrigerator in my basement that has another small freezer, so between the two I make do. My upstairs freezer is mainly filled with fruits and vegetables (and sorbetto or ice cream—yes, we do have treats in our house!). I have our favorites like frozen broccoli and "veggie mix" on hand for nights when I don't have anything in the refrigerator or for snacks like pizza breads or mashed potatoes and mixed veggies. Frozen vegetables are also great to add something extra to your stir fry.

Not only are frozen vegetable convenient, they are also economical. Frozen vegetables, even organic ones, are often less expensive than their fresh counter parts. Since most are frozen very soon after being harvested, frozen veggies don't lose valuable nutrients during travel to the store and are always ripe. Besides buying frozen veggies, I often freeze my own. If I am over zealous at the farmer's market or the grocery store, or if plans change and I find myself left with a lot of extra greens or zucchini, I will freeze them to use for later. This works for a lot of vegetables.

I also freeze extra fruit and herbs. (Don't you hate when you buy fresh herbs and only use a little bit? I never knew what to do with the leftovers. Then I started freezing them. It works great.) Frozen fruits and greens are great for smoothies and when you use them you can often skip the ice. My kids also love making slushies with frozen fruit, like watermelon. They put it in a blender with a little liquid, maybe coconut water or lemonade, and use ice crush mode. For adults, sub out the coconut water for vodka and some lemon juice—frozen watermelon martinis. You can also freeze prepped veggies like chopped onions or leeks. They defrost quickly in a pan, and then you have them on hand all ready when you need them.

My downstairs freezer has frozen meat, soups and other meals. Having frozen meat on hand (if your family eats meat) can be a life saver. Not only when you need something quick, but for when you really don't want to make another trip to the store. Many stores give discounts for buying larger packages of meat (even Whole Foods). I buy the larger package and freeze what I don't need right away. Then I have it on hand when needed. If I need it on the spot, it can be defrosted in the microwave—not ideal but works in a pinch, or if I think about it in advance I can take it out and defrost in refrigerator for the next day.

NOTE

When freezing fruit, a trick is to freeze the fruit pieces flat and separated on a baking sheet covered with parchment paper, once frozen you can put them in a storage bag or other container. This prevents them from sticking together so you don't have to use the whole bag or hit it against the counter or with a hammer to break it apart.)

When you are taking the time to cook, cook extra and freeze it so that you have an easy meal available in the future. Many recipes freeze well, including soups, chili, stews, lasagna, chicken dishes, etc. Remember to label and date what you put in the freezer, so you don't end up with lots of mystery packets that just go to waste. Before freezing, portion out the food how you think you will use it. Individual portions are convenient so that you can just take as many as you need. Having a freezer with prepared dinners can relieve a lot of stress. Not only for when you need something quick, but on a night when your schedule doesn't give you time to cook, you can always add something from your freezer to your weekly meal plan.

Reduce your stress and the amount of time in the kitchen by using tools like a slow cooker and a rice cooker and making the most of your freezer! Simple can be wonderful! When you have less hassle, you really are able to better ENJOY HEALTHY.

CHAPTER 8

MEAL PLANNING

Finally! This is the part you have been waiting for, the "make my life easier" part. You have all the information you need, and now we put it all together in a practical way for you to implement at home.

As stated before, I do believe that with eating healthy "failure to plan is planning to fail." Although meal planning and prep time seem like they are adding things to your already full plate of things to do, they actually save you time, stress, and potentially money in the end.

Meal planning, prepping and cooking is not your only job and therefore should not consume your life! Our main parenting job is to be raising happy, healthy children, not be full-time chefs. Encourage your family to participate in the process and remember you are not being reviewed on your performance so forget about perfection and just do your best.

· Meal Planning Process ·

My meal planning process is relatively easy. You will need your Family Favorites List, your recipes, your family's calendar for the week, a Meal Planning Worksheet, a Shopping List and I highly recommend a clipboard! Although there are a lot of programs and apps out there to help with this process, I still find the old fashion pen and paper way to work best for me. (My goal is to design the ideal meal planning app or software and have someone build it for me, so make sure to sign up for my email alerts so you will know when that happens!)

Starting with dinners, look at the weekly calendar and determine what your meal needs are for the week. Is there a day when you need a slow cooker meal, either because you will be gone all day or the family will need dinner at different times? Is there a night when you have to pack a car picnic because your kids only have the half hour it takes to get from one activity to another to eat? Is there a night when you can cook a meal because you are home in the afternoon and everyone is home for dinner? Do you have time to cook a meal, but need it to be one where all prep can be done in advance? Are you going out one night and just need something for the kids? Do you need a cook-ahead meal or a freezer meal that you can just reheat? You get the idea. Also, take a quick inventory of your fridge, pantry and freezer just to see what you have on hand that may need to be used.

• Get Family Input •

Before you start doing the plan for the week, reach out to your family and ask if there are any requests. If there are, try to incorporate them into the plan. Of course some weeks it is not possible since your child may request a meal that takes too long to prepare or something is out of season. This is a great way to get the family more involved, and looking forward to at least one meal each week! And your family members are great resources; often my kids will remind me of something I haven't made in awhile that we put back into circulation.

You can get your kids even more involved in the prep and cooking as well. If you have older kids, ask them if they would like to cook a meal this week. If your kids are younger, maybe you can find a meal that you can cook together. Look at the calendar and figure out which nights would work best for your kids to help out. Also, use this time to schedule other tasks, such as who will help out with setting the table, or cleaning up each night.

It is important to incorporate everyone's needs into the meal plan without having to cook multiple meals. Since my kids where little and able to eat "real people food," I have made a point of only cooking one meal a night. As I mentioned, there was always PB&J or yogurt or cheese sticks, but I only cooked one meal. When I stopped eating meat, I did not stop cooking meat for my family. We often have meatless meals, but I have learned to cook things that are adaptable. I usually make the meatless version of the chili, or the tacos, or the pasta and then take my portion out before adding the meat or serve the meat on the side.

When grilling, I put my veggie burger or vegetables on the grill with the meat. For recipes like chicken parmesan, I bread the eggplant for the eggplant parm first, and then do the chicken after; although there are two dishes, it is one process. For some of my family's favorite recipes like beef stew, I realize that I am cooking for them and find something easy for myself that night or I might make it on a night I am out. But since that takes such little prep I don't mind. There are many families now that have to accommodate allergies, intolerances or food preferences. Just remember you do not have to be a short order cook. You can accommodate everyone with one meal. That's why the planning time is so helpful.

With your family's input, review your Family Favorites List, and maybe look through the stack of recipes you want to try, to find meals for the remainder of the menu that will fit each night's needs and write them down for the appropriate day in the meal planning worksheet. Consider making double batches to freeze for another time or so that you have left overs for lunches or extras to include in a meal later that week (grilled chicken one night is used for chicken Caesar salad another night or grilled veggies are used for sandwiches one night in pasta later in the week). Don't forget about the things you found in your fridge, freezer or pantry. You can also include ideas like garbage salads or soups ("recipe" is in the appendix), and leftovers. These type of "refrigerator clean out meals" work great at the end of the week so you don't have to hit the store again. Many people like to shop circulars and weekly deals from their stores, and this is a great way to save money and can help with planning. If you see an item that is on special, you can use that to help build your menu for the week by planning a meal around it.

Weekly Meal Plan

	Sunday	Monday	Tuesday	Wednesday	Thursday	Friday	Saturday
Breakfast							
Lunch (Remember leftovers)							
Dinner							
Snacks							

Weekly Meal Plan Worksheet

Also remember that recipes aren't always necessary. When you start filling your refrigerator and pantry with real, healthy food and your family starts to enjoy eating better, it becomes pretty easy to just throw something together like a rice bowl or grilled chicken with broccoli and quinoa. So put those type of easy meals on your plan as well. Our refrigerator is filled with some great condiments that everyone can add to customize their meal—with no recipes or cooking multiple dishes. Just make sure to check the ingredients on the condiments!

Some ideas for condiments and dips are mustard (all types), teriyaki sauce, tamari, herbs and spices (dried and fresh), tahini, nut butters, salad dressing, oils (so many delicious ones), and vinegars. Try a few different ones to see what your family likes.

Once you filled in the worksheet for dinner, pull any recipes needed for that week. Now going through each of the recipes, transfer any ingredients you need to purchase for each recipe to your shopping list.

Some people might have more than one grocery list if you shop at different stores for different things. Having a detailed shopping list will save time and money! If you stick to your list and don't make too many impulse buys, you are getting what you know you will eat in the quantity that you will eat it. (Note: Taking kids or husband shopping with you could completely sabotage this effort!)

Once dinners are done, move onto breakfast, lunch and snacks. I do dinner first so that I can account for leftovers for

TIP

I highly recommend investing your time to create a custom grocery list for the stores where you shop. One day allow a little extra time for your shopping trip and take the time to write down what is in each aisle. Some stores actually have this available if you ask at customer service. You can then create your shopping list based off of this information. Here is an example of the one from my Whole Foods store. Taking the time to do this once will save you a lot of time in the future.

Shopping List: Whole Foods

lunch (or in Paige's case, breakfast, since pasta or mashed potatoes are one of her favorites). When getting your family's input, also ask them for breakfast and lunch ideas. I usually try to get one or two options for each meal and since my kids are older, have the options be things they can make and for lunch pack for themselves. For most, breakfast options are usually the same each week. In my house, it is eggs or smoothies or pb&j or toast with avocado, but sometimes they will request cereal and of course there is always fruit. Although lunches repeat quite often as well, besides from the leftovers, I still ask because maybe they would like a different type of sandwich or something for their salads.

Many people simplify their lives by having their children buy lunch at school, and most think that this is a good healthy option for their children. Please be sure to do some research and really become AWARE of what your kids are being served. The guidelines that are set by the government for school lunches allow a lot of room for interpretation. What I have found in my kids' cafeterias is that the food they are feeding our kids is far from ideal. There are some school districts and private schools that are doing a fabulous job feeding kids real, fresh food, but that is not happening in enough places. As parents we should know what our kids are eating, the best way to do that is to have our kids take their own lunches from home. When you get in the groove of doing it, it will be just as easy (and cost effective and a whole lot healthier) than buying lunch at school.

As for snacks, this includes car food. Knowing what you are going to have to prep and grab on your way to pick up the kids is very beneficial. Again, try to incorporate some fruits like cut up apples and vegetable like carrots and cucumbers with hummus even though grabbing chips or cookies is a lot easier. When I am home before pick up and I have time, I have made my kids nachos with salsa for a car ride. I covered them in tin foil to keep them warm. Another favorite of my kids is fresh popcorn (with maple syrup and salt, our favorite; just remember to have some wipes).

Go through the same process with breakfast, lunch and snacks of adding anything you need to your grocery list, and don't forget to add any staples you have run out of during the week. I keep a list on my refrigerator door so when someone uses the last of something they can write it down and I can just add these items to my shopping list. (My kids and husband are still trying to get the hang of this!) There are also apps for your phone where multiple family members can add things to the list.

So, I bet you were wondering what that clipboard was for... Well, although you may feel a little geeky in the store, I recommend putting all the recipes for the week, your meal plan and your shopping list on the clipboard and taking it with you to the store. First, you can stand the clipboard up in the shopping cart for convenience (if you don't have a kid in there and if you do, they can hold it.) Second, when you go to buy that item you put on the list for a recipe and you don't remember what it was for or how much you need... the recipes are right there. Third, you have everything organized for the week.

Ideally, you would only have to shop once for the week but we all know that is unrealistic. We run out of things, or need to buy something for a meal later in the week that we either forgot or wanted to buy fresh, but this process will minimize the trips to the store and shorten the "fill in" trips later in the week.

· Scheduling and Prepping

Now that we have planned, it is important to schedule time to execute! I tell clients to figure out when works best for them to plan and then shop and to actually put it into their calendars. Make appointments in your calendar for prep! I know it sounds silly, but if it is in your calendar, you have made time and committed to it. This is also often recommended for exercise or anything else that you could easily blow off. If time is allotted in your calendar, you also have less stress about how you will get it all done.

As an example, here is a typical week for me and my family for meal planning, shopping and prep. I usually try to start the process on Saturday, sometimes it happens Sunday morning. I print out our calendar for the week, a meal plan and a shopping list. (I have a folder with meal plans and shopping lists on hand to make it easier—print once, use for weeks!) I ask my family if they have any requests for the week. Since my 15-year-old Emily wants to be a chef, I see if she has some time in her schedule to cook dinner one night and what she would like to make (reminding her that clean up comes with cooking!)

I check the refrigerator to see if there is anything that needs to be used. Then I sit down and fill in the menu for the week. I make a shopping list off of the recipes (ingredients) and our "ran out of" list. While making the list, I check the pantry and the fridge/freezer to see if I have any items on hand. Sunday is my shopping day. I go to the store, get what I need and then come home to do some prep. I wash and prep greens and veggies, maybe make a soup or steam some greens or do any of the prep work I can do for the week with the food before I put it away. As long as the cutting board is out, might as well chop and prep as many veggies as I can! Then I store them in zip-lock bags or air tight containers. I may even make a dinner for later in the week if I have time or make some salads for lunches or overnight oats or pre-measured smoothies for breakfast. These are real time savers during the week. During farmer's market season this changes a bit, because I go to the market on Sunday mornings first before the store and given what I find there I might make some changes to my plan and shopping list.

I know, it sounds like I spend my whole Sunday shopping and prepping. Some Sundays I do spend a good amount of time on preparing for the week, but the more time I spend on Sunday, the less time I have to spend during the busy weekdays. Since I work from home, I can often fit in some planned prep during the week and I try to schedule that as well. Also, this is what works for my family and me. Sunday morning my girls have religious school so I can hit the farmer's market and shop while they are there (and when they don't have school, as teenagers they can sleep until at least noon!). During the fall, I can prep in the kitchen while watching the game with my husband. I know others that would rather spend the time during the week shopping and prepping, or who wait to find out what is in their CSA box or on sale before they plan for the week. Do what works best for you. Just make sure to have a plan and schedule time to shop and prep. For me, Sunday works best because I usually just plan for Monday-Friday and then wing the weekends.

•

IN SUMMARY

Living in a time where celebrity chefs are as famous as movie stars, and we constantly see them make delicious home cooked meals "easily" on television, it is easy to feel the pressure to serve restaurant-quality food every night. Remember, they have people who do all the shopping, prep and clean up for them, plus many have years of experience and of course are professionally trained chefs!

Your job as a parent is to feed your family healthy, not to dazzle their taste buds every night. (Honestly, most kids I know don't really care as much about what the food is, just as long as it is there and tastes good.) Find some meals your family enjoys, do a makeover if necessary and keep it simple. It is about the quality of the meals and the time together, not the variety or if it is gourmet. You do not have to reinvent the wheel every week. For most families the schedule of activities is pretty consistent from week to week, so find some meal plans that work and reuse them. My husband tells me how growing up at his house Monday was Meatloaf night, Tuesday was pasta night, etc; every week the same thing. (OK that's a little boring, but you get the idea.)

Good healthy food does not need to be complicated or overly time consuming. (Don't forget: the goal is to ENJOY HEALTHY!) Remember to get your kids involved, let them make or help make their breakfast and/or lunch the night before. Have them cook with you in the kitchen. Many schools do not offer home economics anymore, so it is up to us as parents to teach them the basics, like how to read a recipe, measure ingredients, boil water, cook pasta, etc. It took me a while to realize that I had to teach my kids these basic things that we learned in school.

We are also teaching our kids healthy habits. Most schools teach brief nutrition during health class, most of which is dated. They teach about reading the numbers on the label and about calories, but not about eating real food. Luckily, celebrities are taking on the cause. People like Jamie Oliver with his *Food Revolution* are trying to get food education for every child and Dr. Katz with his T*urn the Tide Foundation*, that includes programs like *Nutrition Detectives*^{TM}, a nutritional education program for elementary school kids, are getting the important information to kids at an early age. Some schools are growing gardens and teaching the kids where their food comes from as well as teaching them how to eat healthy. This is a great trend, but as parents, we need to take on the responsibility of teaching our kids healthy habits ourselves.

I know this may seem like a lot to take in, and depending on where you are starting your journey, it may seem a little overwhelming. Take a breath and remember to strive for progress not perfection. Take baby steps by setting realistic goals. And cut yourself some slack! I don't even follow my rules all the time! I have weeks that get out of control or away from me, and I love the occasional indulgence —we are human and as I have said deprivation is not enjoyable. So remember the 80/20 or 90/10 rule, you do not have to be "perfect" all the time!

Raising kids is a tough job; feeding your family healthy meals shouldn't be. Take it slow and figure out what works for your family. Get back to basics. Eat more plants. Drink more water. Little by little, you incorporate small changes and they become your new normal. As a Busy Mom, your life is full. Feeding your family healthy meals does not have to be a burden. In fact, it will lighten your load. When you start eating better, you will start feeling better. More energy to get you through the busy days!

This book is a guide to help you create meals with less stress, less time, and less money. Hopefully it has taught you that it is worth the small investment of your time upfront to free up the crazed "what's for dinner" dilemma every night. Small changes in how you operate can make every day go smoother and be a more pleasant experience for you and your family.

Using the **ADD, AWARE, ADJUST** and **ENJOY**™ method will allow your family to ENJOY HEALTHY!

APPENDIX

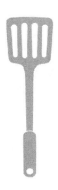

WORKSHEETS

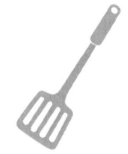

Throughout the text, I share several tools to help you keep on track with your journey of ADD, AWARE, ADJUST, ENJOY™ method. I've included them here in larger format, and you may also download them on my website: http://www.enjoyhealthy.me.

Family Food List

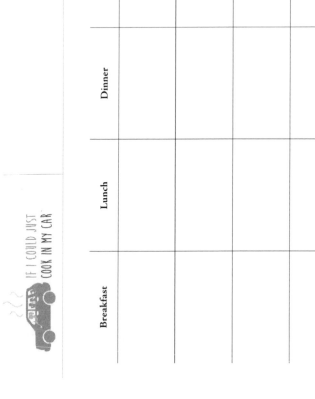

Breakfast	Lunch	Dinner	Sides	Snacks

Notes

enjoy healthy

© 2015 *If I Could Just Cook In My Car* • enjoyhealthy.me

IF I COULD JUST
COOK IN MY CAR

Sanderson Family Food List

Breakfast	Lunch	Dinner	Sides/Snacks
Nutella® with strawberries or Bananas	Wraps - Chicken or Turkey	Stuffed Shells	Kale chips
Eggs	PB&J	Chili	Salad
PB&J	Soup	Burgers	Mashed potatoes
Toast	Peanut Butter with apple and Pretzels	Chicken/eggplant "Parm"	Sweet potato chips
Waffles	Hummus and Veggies	Roast Chicken	Whole sweet potatoes
Pancakes	Fried Rice	Quesadillas	Veggies - roasted, steamed
Smoothies	Pasta Salad	Fajitas/tacos - veggie, meat, fish	Spinach and mushrooms sautéed
Granola and yogurt	Chicken nuggets	Thai lettuce wraps	Quinoa with veggies
Toast with avocado	Salad	Spring rolls	"Fries"
Cereal	Pasta	Mussels	Popcorn - maple, smart pop
Oatmeal - overnight or instant	Rice with cucumber and avocado	Fish: pan seared/in parchment	Hummus and veggies
Fruit		Grilled veggie sandwiches	Guacamole with veggies
		Chicken Cesar salad with garlic pita	Nachos with guacamole and salsa
		Potato Bar	Corn on the cob
		Turkey/veggie chili	
		Pulled chicken	
		Pizza breads	
		Shepard's pie	
		Hot dogs and/or hamburgers	
		Buffalo broc/cauliflower and wings	
		Zucchini pasta with pesto or other sauce	
		Pasta with Alfredo or veggie sauce	
		Turkey meatball subs	

Notes

enjoy healthy

EXAMPLE

IF I COULD JUST COOK IN MY CAR

Weekly Meal Plan

	Sunday	Monday	Tuesday	Wednesday	Thursday	Friday	Saturday
Breakfast							
Lunch (Remember leftovers)							
Dinner							
Snacks							

enjoy healthy

IF I COULD JUST COOK IN MY CAR

Shopping List: Whole Foods

Fruits and vegetables	Bulk
Hummus/tortillas/cheese	Bars/ Canned Fruit/ Applesauce
Cereal/Non-Dairy Milk	Water/Paper Products
Chips/Salsa/Rice Cakes	Cookies/Crackers/ juice/soup
Baking/Chocolate	Beans/rice/pasta
Condiments/asian/oil/vinegar	Frozen
Refrig	Meat
Bread/Deli	Other

enjoy healthy

RECIPES

My daughter Paige suggested that I include some of our family recipes, so here they are. Just a note about my recipes: I personally eat a plant-based diet. I eat fish, but I don't eat meat, and try to avoid dairy, eggs and gluten. My family does eat all of that stuff but to make it so that I don't have to cook multiple times, many of my recipes use ingredients to accommodate me. Feel free to substitute whatever works for your family, I won't be offended if you use cow's milk or eggs because that's what you had on hand or what your family prefers. I am a throw it together type of gal, so substitutions and modifications sound great to me!

Remember to check ingredients on things like stocks or broths, breadcrumbs, tomato paste or other prepared ingredients for unwanted things like MSG or unneeded sugar and upgrade ingredients where you can!

Some ingredients in the recipes might be unfamiliar, so here is a brief introduction:

COCONUT WATER: No to be confused with creamy coconut milk, coconut water is the clear liquid tapped from the center of the coconut. The clear slightly sweet liquid contains easily digestible carbs, electrolytes and lots of potassium which is why some like to use it as a sports drink and why I use it in my post workout smoothies.

CHIA SEEDS: Yes these are the same little black seeds we used to spread over the ceramic "chia pets" to watch the "hair" grow. Who knew that years later they would be such a popular super-food! They are a good plant based source of Omega 3's, anti-oxidants, dietary fiber and protein and contain minerals like calcium and iron. Because they absorb water and plump up they create a feeling of fullness and are a great thickener. I always add them to my smoothies among other things.

GROUND FLAX SEEDS: My understanding is that your body cannot process whole flax seeds, so when incorporating flaxseed into your diet it is best to use ground. Similar to Chia Seeds they are a good source of Omega 3, protein and dietary fiber. They also absorb water to help fill you up and they have the added benefit of helping to keep you regular (just make sure to drink enough water!) Again I add to smoothies, and among other things, use it in recipes as an egg replacer. For each egg you want to replace in a recipe, combine 1 Tablespoon of ground flax and 3 Table-spoons of warm water, let this mixture sit for about 15 minutes to thicken and get goopy then add to recipe instead of eggs.

HEMP SEEDS: My love of these little nutty seeds started when I was looking for a powerhouse plant protein sources. Instead of using a hemp powder, I just started using the yummy seeds. A good source of easily digestible plant based protein. They contain essential fatty acids, minerals, and fiber. Yup, I throw these in smoothies too! I also sprinkle on my salad, and add to my granola or nut ball recipes.

COCAO: No I did not spell it wrong! The difference between cocoa and cocao is that cocao is made by cold –pressing the raw cocao bean thus maintaining all the good stuff like enzymes. Where cocoa is made from beans that have been roasted at high heat, that can destroy the good stuff. Cacao is high in antioxi-dant and nutrients including magnesium. You can use it as a substitute for unsweetened cocoa powder in recipes to get a healthy chocolate fix.

COCONUNT OIL: Recently coconut oil has gotten a lot of press for having health benefits. Many claims have been made, but for me the jury is still out so I don't currently recommend eating it by itself in high quantities! I like to cook with it because of its taste and because it has a high smoke point. Smoke point is the temperature where oil decomposes and potentially toxic byproducts are formed. So when cooking with high heat, coconut oil is a great option. Coconut oil will be solid at room temperature and turn to a liquid when heated. Make sure to buy virgin or unrefined coconut oil.

NUTRITIONAL YEAST: Usually sold in the baking aisle in a canister, these yellow flakes' "cheesy" taste makes them ideal for adding a cheese flavor without the dairy. Often used in vegan cooking, it also packs a nutritional punch. A great vegan source of B12 it is also a complete protein. I sprinkle it on everything from popcorn to soup and use it in recipes instead of cheese.

QUINOA: Technically a seed not a grain, quinoa is a complete protein. Which makes it a great source of non-animal protein! Quinoa does not have to be soaked before use, but does need to be rinsed very well to remove the bitter coating of saponins. It can be eaten as a side, main course or added to soups, stews, or salads.

NATURAL "REAL" MAPLE SYRUP: Yes, I am a maple syrup fanatic! I love the stuff, but the REAL stuff not the high fructose corn syrup pancake syrup. Pure maple syrup that comes from trees not only tastes amazing, but has nutritional benefits as well. It contains minerals like zinc and manganese and antioxidants. I know it can be a little pricey, but you don't need to use a lot to get the health benefits or sweetness. Although it is a healthier alternative, remember it is still sugar!

SMOOTHIES

· Smoothies ·

There are lots of smoothie recipes out there, but it is also fun and easy to create your own. There are no wrong answers. Start with a liquid base, add greens, fruits, maybe some superfoods/nut butters and blend. As for amounts, I usually use about 1 cup of liquid, 1½ cups of fruit and 1 cup or so of greens. Play with the amounts, maybe you like more liquid or more greens and less fruit. Sometimes I make smoothies and use no greens. Those are more like treats for me.

You can add ice to your smoothie, or use frozen fruits or greens. Remember those greens and berries you froze because you had too many and didn't want them to go to waste? Throw them in your smoothie!

Smoothies should last in the refrigerator for 2 days (depending on ingredients). If you want to make some ahead of time or make extra, just keep it in a sealed container and shake before drinking. Personally I like to make them fresh since I usually put in my trilogy of 1Tbs each of hemp seed, ground flax and chia seeds. Chia seeds, when left in liquid overnight, make a great pudding, but I don't love the chunks in my smoothie! Clean up from smoothies is easy, as long as you clean the blender right after you make the smoothie!

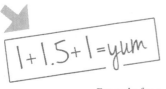

Formula for a delicious and healthy smoothie

Here are some ideas for smoothie ingredients and a few of my personal favorites...

Liquid Base	Main Ingredient	Super Food
Water	1 cup leafy greens: Spinach, kale, Romaine, swiss chard	Super foods or protein sources: chia seeds, flax seed (ground), cinnamon, hemp seeds, almond butter, coconut oil, cocao
Coconut water (especially good after a workout)		
Unsweetened coconut, almond or other nut milk	1 1/2 cups fruit: Banana, Berries, Avocado, Pear, Apple	
Unsweetened fruit juice (might want to dilute)		

Here are my go-to smoothies:

• Post work-out Smoothie •

* ½ cup coconut water
* ½ cup water
* 1 banana
* ½ cup frozen blueberries
* handful (approximately ½-1 cup) of frozen greens
* 1 Tbs each of chia seeds, hemp seeds and ground flaxseed

• Chocolate Banana Smoothie •

* 1 cup unsweetened almond milk (*Make your own or check those ingredients – no carrageenan – what is that anyway?*)
* 1 banana
* 1-2 Tbs almond butter
* 1Tbs raw cocao powder (not processed cocoa powder)
* Ice
* Optional 1 Tbs each of chia seeds, hemp seeds and ground flaxseed

• Fruit Smoothie •

* 1 cup unsweetened almond milk
* 1 banana
* ½ cup strawberries (fresh or frozen)
* ½ cup of blueberries (fresh or frozen)
* Ice
* Optional 1 Tbs each of chia seeds, hemp seeds and ground flaxseed

I personally don't eat dairy, but if you do, feel free to use regular milk for your base or add yogurt to your smoothie. My kids make the following smoothie for breakfast:

• Emily's Special •

* ½ cup coconut water or orange juice
* 1 banana
* ½-1 cup berries (*usually frozen strawberries/blueberries*
* 1 5-6oz container Greek yogurt (* *You can buy sweetened yogurt, but another option is to buy plain and use honey or maple syrup to sweeten to liking.*)

BAKED KALE CHIPS

I know you might not believe me, but chances are your family will like these! Just remember to be patient with them and check on them often so they don't burn.

Ingredients

* 1 bunch kale (Lacinato or Dinosaur Kale is my favorite)
* 1 Tbs olive oil
* ¼ tsp fine sea salt
* You can also add toppings like parmesan cheese, nutritional yeast, garlic powder, etc.

Directions

1. Preheat oven to 300 degrees. Line 1 or 2 baking sheets with parchment paper

2. Wash kale and spin or pat dry. Cut away the center spine of each leaf and discard the spine (unless you want to save them for juicing or finely chopping to add to some other recipe). Cut or rip the leaves into pieces approximately 3-4 inches by 3-4 inches.

3. Place kale, oil and salt in a large bowl and toss. Make sure to cover each kale piece thoroughly.

4. Arrange the pieces in a single layer on the baking sheets and then bake until crisp, about 25 minutes. Check kale every 10 minutes or so and turn them over every so often so they don't burn.

The kale chips will stay crisp and fresh for up to 1 week stored in a sealed container or bag.

Note: These are really fun and easy to make even without a recipe. Just toss kale with oil put them on the pan and sprinkle with whatever you think would taste good. Start with just salt and then have fun! You can even make them sweet by adding a bit of maple syrup when you toss them in the oil.

MAPLE SYRUP POPCORN

I came up with this idea years ago after I had Kettle Corn for the first time during college. Trying to recreate it in my dorm room I popped some corn in my hot air popper and drizzled maple syrup on top. Although it wasn't exactly Kettle Corn, it was REALLY GOOD!

I now have a Whirly Pop which is an invaluable tool if your family loves popcorn like mine does! We use coconut oil since it can tolerate the high heat needed to make popcorn.

Ingredients

* Bowl of freshly popped popcorn
* Pure maple syrup
* Sea salt
* Nutritional yeast (optional)

Directions

1. Drizzle maple syrup over popcorn shaking bowl to make sure all kernels get some of the goodness.
2. Sprinkle with sea salt and yeast, if using, or any other topping you may like.
3. Enjoy, but make sure to have some wet towels available; this can get a little sticky.

BBQ BROCCOLI/CAULIFLOWER "WINGS"

The first time I made this dish was for a Super Bowl party. I have to say everyone really liked it and didn't even care that it was cauliflower! After having a version made with broccoli at a restaurant, I started making it with both broccoli and cauliflower – although Paige prefers just broccoli!

Ingredients
* 4 cups of broccoli and/ or cauliflower
* Batter for "wings"
* Sauce

Batter
* 1 cup oat flour
* 1 cup almond milk
* 2 Tbs nutritional yeast
* ½ tsp garlic powder
* ½ tsp onion powder
* ½ tsp sea salt

Sauce
* ¼ cup hot sauce (I use Frank's red hot)
* ¼ cup bbq sauce
* 1 Tbs coconut oil
* 2 Tbs maple syrup

Directions

1. Preheat oven to 450 degrees. Cover a baking sheet with parchment paper.

2. Prepare broccoli/cauliflower by cutting into "wings". For the broccoli you can just use the "trees" or you can also cut the stems into coins and use them too (I peel the stems if using).

3. In a bowl combine the flour, milk, nutritional yeast, garlic powder, onion powder and sea salt. Use a whisk to mix well.

4. Dip the veggies in the batter to coat, and then put on prepared baking sheet. Place in oven and cook until crispy, about 20 minutes.

5. While veggies are cooking make the sauce. Combine all the ingredients in a pot and heat until warm and coconut oil has melted (adjust the sauce's spice according to your family's taste .) When veggies are crispy, pour sauce over to coat, then put back in oven for an additional 8-10 minutes .

6. Remove from oven and serve! My family likes them with ranch dressing!

GARBAGE SALAD

This is the way I usually eat salad. I throw a bunch of cut up stuff in a bowl over lettuce and eat. Or I throw a bunch of stuff in a bowl and use my salad chopper to create an easy chopped salad.

Here are some ideas for salad ingredients.

Directions

1. Start with GREENS!! (Feel free to combine a few or all!)
   * Arugula
   * Spinach
   * Spring Mix
   * Romaine
   * Baby Romaine
   * Kale (make sure to cut up into small pieces)
   * Mesclun Mix
   * Any green leafy thing

2. Then add whatever is in your fridge
   * Cooked Tempeh
   * Beans
   * Nuts and Seeds
   * Raisins
   * Berries
   * Avocado
   * Olives
   * Tomatoes
   * Broccoli
   * Cauliflower
   * Mushrooms
   * Cooked or Raw Beets
   * Cooked Sweet Potato
   * Artichoke Hearts
   * Celery
   * Carrots
   * Radishes
   * Cucumbers
   * Quinoa
   * Brown Rice
   * Chicken Breast
   * Turkey Meat
   * Cheese
   * Steak

My favorite dressing is just olive oil, lemon juice and sea salt. I have also experimented with adding miso paste and nutritional yeast or both to the dressing and both are yummy!

Be careful of bottled dressings, make sure to check ingredients. Best to make your own using oil, something acidic tasting like lemon/lime juice or vinegar and some seasonings like salt and pepper, cumin, cayenne, basil... You can also always add maple syrup for sweetness or mustard for flavor.

GARBAGE SOUP

I love soup! So easy to make, no recipe needed. Here are the basics on how to make soup.

Directions

1. **CHOP VEGGIES** – Any you have on hand. I usually start with onions, carrots and celery and if I am in the mood, garlic. Then I add whatever I have in my fridge that looks good – mushrooms, broccoli, greens, zucchini, sweet potatoes, daikon radish, kohlrabi squash.

2. **SAUTE** – Heat a stockpot and add a little oil, enough to coat the bottom. I usually use coconut or olive. Then add the veggies and sauté. I always do the garlic first, then onions until they are translucent. Next, I add the other ingredients according to how long they take to cook: harder veggies that take longer to cook first, quicker cooking veggies last. (Don't add the greens now, they go in at the very end). You can also add in spices, or hearty herbs here if you like.

3. **ADD LIQUID** – Once the vegetables are softened you can add the stock or water. When using store bought vegetable stock, just make sure to check the label for sugar or any other unwanted ingredients except veggies Make sure to cover the veggies with the liquid; you can always add more liquid later if needed.

4. **COVER AND SIMMER** – Cook time will depend on what vegetable you have used and how soft you want them. I usually start checking to see if the veggies are soft enough around 20 minutes.

5. **ADD GREENS** – Once the soup is to your liking you can add the greens. They will cook quickly.

6. **SEASON TO TASTE** – Add salt and pepper or other spices or herbs to taste.

OTHER OPTIONS – Puree some or all of your soup after it is done cooking. Add cooked beans or uncooked lentils to the soup before you cover and simmer. Puree and add some non-dairy milk for a creamy soup.

Make a big pot, put it in the refrigerator and eat it for lunch, dinner, snack… Soup is really filling and satisfying.

ARUGULA QUINOA SALAD

This salad is always a bit hit. I think it is from the sweetness of the grapes and the crunch of the pine nuts. You can change the fruit, greens or nuts, or add in more veggies to your liking. The idea is using a grain in your salad to bulk it up. You can also add a protein (although quinoa is a great source of protein) like grilled chicken, or shrimp.

My sister in law Julie taught me how to cook quinoa perfectly every time and I share it with you in this recipe. The ratio of liquid to quinoa is probably different than what the bag says or you see other places. I like to use vegetable broth when making quinoa to add flavor, but water works just as well.

Ingredients

* 1 cup dry quinoa
* 1 ½ cups vegetable broth or water
* approx. 6 cup baby arugula
* ½ cup halved green or red grapes
* 1/4 cup toasted pine nuts
* 2 small scallions sliced

Dressing

* 2 lime or 1 lemon, juiced
* 4 tsp extra virgin olive oil
* 2 tsp maple syrup
* Sea salt
* Black pepper

Directions

1. Rinse the quinoa well, then put it in a pot with the vegetable broth or water. Bring to a boil. Once at a boil cover, reduce heat and simmer for 14 minutes (I know it's a weird number but it's magical for quinoa). Without lifting the lid, remove from heat and let sit 14 minutes. Remove lid and fluff with a fork. Let cool.

2. While quinoa is cooking, toast the pine nuts in a dry pan until golden. Let cool.

3. Whisk the ingredients for the dressing until they come together, seasoning to taste. Set to the side.

4.   Mix ingredients in a bowl, and toss with dressing.

THAI CHICKEN LETTUCE WRAPS

This is an assemble your own dinner with a lot of components – pick and choose what your family will like and maybe add something new. The original inspiration came from the Wraps at the Cheesecake Factory. I searched on line for recipes and over time have simplified and altered to fit my families liking and made it easier for me!

THAI CHICKEN SATAYS

Ingredients

* 1 lb boneless skinless chicken breast cut into strips
* 1/4 cup tamari or soy sauce *tamari is gluten free soy sauce*
* 2 TBS fresh lime juice
* 2 cloves garlic – minced
* 1 tsp grated fresh ginger
* 3/4 tsp red pepper flakes (optional)
* 2 TBS water
* 4 green onions chopped into small pieces
* Bamboo skewers (10-12 inches)

Directions

Note: I put the chicken on the skewers before I marinate just to save me a step later, but you can marinate the chicken first and then thread on to skewers. Either way make sure to soak the skewers for about 20 minutes in water first to help prevent them from burning.

1.   Combine soy sauce, lime juice, garlic, ginger and red pepper flakes (if using), green onion and water in a small bowl and whisk together.

2. Thread chicken on to soaked skewers and place in a large shallow baking dish. Pour marinade over chicken and refrigerate for at least 30 minutes. If marinade does not completely cover chicken, rotate while marinating. (Remember, you can also marinate chicken before putting on skewers)

3. Place the skewers on grill and brush with marinade. Cook using indirect medium for 6-8 minutes until chicken is cooked through, turning hallway through grilling.
   I grill my skewers outside on my as grill using indirect medium, but you can also cook them in your oven using the broiler or on a stove top grill.

BEAN SPROUTS

* 1 package fresh bean sprouts (*Can use canned sprouts but check ingredient list for added salt and adjust accordingly)
* 1 tsp raw sesame seeds
* 1 Tbs tamari or soy sauce
* 1 Tbs sesame oil
  *These are guidelines for the sesame oil and tamari, season to taste. My family doesn't like the taste of sesame oil so I either leave it out or I use less.

Directions

1. Toast sesame seeds briefly in a dry frying pan making sure not to burn. Add other ingredients and sauté until sprouts have softened.

2. Put in refrigerator to cool.

NOODLES

The original recipe calls for making Thai Curry noodles, which are delicious, but labor intensive. So I switched to just using plain brown rice vermicelli noodles, cooked according to directions.. The dipping sauces replace the noodle seasoning.

MARINATED CUCUMBERS

* 1 large cucumber, seeded
* Rice vinegar
* Water
* Sugar

1. Make marinade by putting vinegar, water, and sugar in a small pot and stirring until sugar is dissolved. Let cool. (*This marinade is very similar to sushi vinegar and you can use it as a substitute.)
2. Cut cucumbers into small bite size pieces, place in a bowl and cover with marinade. Mix to blend, cover and put in refrigerator to marinate. The longer you let them marinate, the better.

TO ASSEMBLE WRAPS

* Head of butter or Boston lettuce
* Chicken Satays
* Sprouts
* Cucumbers
* Noodles
* Dipping Sauces – there are recipes on line for original sauces. (We use bottled peanut sauce, tamari sauce and Anne's Teriyaki Sauce.

Directions

1. Remove full leaves from head of lettuce, wash and dry and lay on a platter.
2. Put out the fillings and the sauces and let your family make their own wraps!

....

SLOW-COOKER BEEF STEW

I prep everything for this stew the night before by cutting the veggies and measuring out the other ingredients. In the morning, all I have to do is quickly brown the meat and add everything to the pot.

Ingredients

* 2 lbs beef stew meat (cut into bite-sized pieces)
* 1 TBS olive oil
* veggies – chopped (*This is just a basic list feel free to add others)*
    * 1 medium onion
    * 3 celery ribs
    * 4-5 large carrots peeled
    * 1 cup baby bella mushrooms
    * 4-5 red potatoes or one sweet potato (cut into bite size pieces)

* 2 – 3 cloves crushed and minced garlic
* 6 oz tomato paste
* 32 oz beef broth
* 2 Tbs Worcestershire Sauce
* Herbs - I usually use 1 tsp of both dried parsley and oregano , but you could also use rosemary, thyme or herbs de provence. Experiment with types and quantities.
* Salt and pepper to taste

Directions

1. Prep all ingredients, chopping veggies and making sure that beef is cut into bite size pieces. Remember you can add as many different veggies as you like, just make sure you have enough liquid to fully cover them all.

2. Optional – I like to brown the beef before adding other ingredients, but it is not necessary. My slow cooker has an insert that can be put on the stove so there are no extra dishes to brown the beef. If you choose to brown beef, heat the olive oil, add beef and briefly brown on all sides.

3. Add veggies, potatoes, garlic, tomato paste, beef broth, Worcestershire sauce, herbs and salt and pepper to the beef in the slow cooker. Cover and cook on low for 10

hours or high for 6-7 hours until beef and veggies are cooked and tender.

I serve the stew over mashed potatoes; you can also serve over pasta or with a loaf of yummy crusty bread.

If you like a thicker stew, about 30 minutes before serving, mix ¼ cup of flour and ½ cup of water in a small bowl and add to stew to thicken. Replace lid and let cook for the final 30 minutes.

SLOW-COOKER BBQ
PULLED CHICKEN SANDWICHES

This can actually be as easy as combining a jar of your favorite BBQ sauce with some chicken breasts in the slow cooker. and turning the cooker on. In this version, I have doctored up the jar of BBQ sauce a little. As always feel free to adjust to your family's tastes. If your family likes it really sweet, then add more sugar and the sweeter balsamic dressing.. If you prefer a tangier sauce, add a tangy Italian dressing and even throw in a bit of hot pepper sauce!

Serve the pulled chicken on rolls in a sandwich or it can be eaten over rice or mashed potatoes! It is even better as leftovers and freezes pretty well – so make a double batch!

Ingredients

* 2 pounds of chicken breast
* 1 cup of your favorite BBQ sauce (*Remember to read that label on your BBQ sauce!)
* ½ cup of balsamic vinaigrette or Italian dressing
* 1 Tbs of Worstershire sauce
* 1 Tbs of mustard (optional)
* ¼ cup of brown sugar
* Rolls

Directions

1. Place chicken breast in slow cooker.
2. Whisk together the rest of the ingredients in a small bowl. Taste and adjust to suit your liking.
3. Pour sauce over chicken and cover. Cook on high for about 4 hours or until chicken is tender and can easily be "shredded" with a fork.

4. Using 2 forks "pull" or shred the chicken. Mix the shredded chicken back in with the sauce in the slow cooker and let cook another 10-15 minutes.

5. Serve on buns, with a veggie of course! We usually make coleslaw to go with it!

PAIGE'S PEANUT BUTTER CUPS

My daughter Paige makes these when she wants a chocolate treat. She originally made them in a Pyrex dish, but it was hard to cut. So she came up with the idea of using mini cupcake tins lined with cupcake wrappers. She also recommends using a "mini ice cream scoop", aka a melon baller, to put the ingredients in the "cups".

You can enjoy occasional treats and still ENJOY HEALTHY. When making a treat like this at home you have control of what goes into them. Check the ingredients and choose chocolate chips that are real chocolate (or buy a bar of good chocolate and cut it up) and use peanut butter or other nut butter that is just ground nuts.

These can be made with your chocolate of choice or you can mix chocolates. Paige also wanted to include a version without peanut butter. She is always concerned for those with allergies.

Ingredients

* 1 cup of chocolate chips (or chopped chocolate); you will need 1/3 cup for the bottom layer and 2/3 cup for the top. Paige likes to use 1/3 semi sweet, milk or dark on the bottom and 2/3 cup of white chocolate chips for the top
* 1/3 cup of peanut butter (or nut butter of your choice)

Directions

1. Prepare a 12 cup mini cupcake tin by lining each cup with a cupcake wrapper.
2. Place 1/3 cup of the chocolate you want to use for the bottom layer in a microwave safe bowl. Microwave for about a minute then carefully take out. (Bowl will be hot.) Mix the chocolate with a fork or a spoon. If not melted, return to microwave for a bit longer but be careful not to

burn it. (Time will vary depending on your microwave, try 30 seconds at a time to start)

3. Fill each cupcake wrapper with ½ a melon ball scoop (about 1 ½ teaspoons if you don't have a scoop) of the melted chocolate. Shake the tin a little so that the chocolate evenly covers the bottom of each cup.

4. Place in freezer for 15 minutes or until hardened.

5. Scoop ½ of melon ball scoop (again about 1 ½ tsp) of peanut butter on top the top of the hardened chocolate.

6. Place 2/3 cup of the chocolate you want to use on the top in a microwave safe bowl, repeat process to melt chocolate and scoop 1 melon ball scoop on top of the peanut butter. Again, shaking the tray to even out the chocolate.

7. Place in refrigerator to harden. When chocolate is hardened, candies are ready to eat.

Note: Peanut butter cups get pretty hard in the refrigerator so you might want to let them sit out a bit to soften before eating!

NUT—FREE VERSION: Replace the middle peanut/nut butter layer with white chocolate. Paige's trick is to mix semisweet and white chips together for the top layer, topping with chocolate chips to make them look fancy. Adjust the amount of chocolate as needed to make the number of layers and thickness you desire.

WHIPPED CREAM AND BERRIES

This is a very easy go-to dessert in my house. Emily makes really great whipped cream, and homemade is so much better than canned! It tastes better and you can control the sweetness and the ingredients going into it. (Just because it is a dessert doesn't mean you shouldn't use upgraded ingredients like organic cream. You can even experiment with flavors like adding cocao powder for chocolate whipped cream.)

The secret to really great whipped cream is to start with a cold bowl. Put the bowl in the freezer for a little bit before you get started. Of course, be careful when taking out a metal bowl- you don't want your fingers to stick!

Ingredients

* 1 cup heavy whipping cream
* 1 -2 Tbs sugar
* splash of vanilla extract (Emily's secret ingredient)
* washed and cleaned berries

Directions

1. Pour cold cream into prepared bowl and whisk by hand or with an electric mixer until becomes stiff.
2. Add 1 Tbs sugar and splash of vanilla *(This is where you would add other flavors as well)*
3. Continue to mix until combined.
4. Add more sugar to taste.
5. Place berries in a bowl and top with whipped cream! Enjoy! Refrigerate any extra whipped cream, covered.

You can also make non-dairy whipped cream using coconut cream, which is the solid stuff in a can of whole fat coconut milk. Just put the can in the refrigerator overnight. In the morning, take it out and turn upside down. Pour off liquid "milk" on top – you can keep the milk to use in coffee or smoothies. Take the solid stuff that is left and put it in a cold bowl. Whip as above until fluffy "whipped cream" consistency. Then add sweetener and vanilla and whip to combine.

ABOUT THE AUTHOR

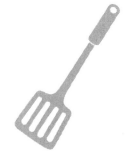

After making substantial changes in her diet and lifestyle, Lisa decided to become a Certified Health Coach through the Institute for Integrative Nutrition. It's now her passion to help others ENJOY HEALTHY. Realizing most of her clients were Busy Moms who not only had their own health to think about, but their family's as well, Lisa decided to share her process of how she overcame the frustration of feeding her family healthy. Lisa knows you and your family can ENJOY HEALTHY too.

Lisa Sanderson has her B.S.B.A. from Washington University in St. Louis, her M.B.A. from Georgetown, and worked in Brand Management before going full time for her M.O.M. from daughter's Emily and Paige.